Cancer Detection

UICC Monograph Series · Volume 4

Cancer Detection

Prepared by the Cancer Detection Committee
of the Commission on Cancer Control

Second, Revised Edition

Edited by A. J. Phillips

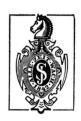

Springer-Verlag Berlin Heidelberg New York 1974

ALEXANDER J. PHILLIPS PH. D.
National Cancer Institute, 25 Adelaide Street East, Toronto 1, Canada

ISBN 3-540-06976-3 2. Auflage Springer-Verlag Berlin Heidelberg New York
ISBN 0-387-06976-3 2nd edition Springer-Verlag New York Heidelberg Berlin

ISBN 3-540-04006-4 1. Auflage Springer-Verlag Berlin · Heidelberg · New York
ISBN 0-387-04006-4 1st edition Springer-Verlag New York · Heidelberg · Berlin

Library of Congress Cataloging in Publication Data. International Union Against Cancer. Commission on Cancer Control. Cancer Detection Committee. Cancer detection. (UICC monograph series, v. 4) Bibliography: p. 1. Cancer-Diagnosis. I. Title. II. Series: International Union Against Cancer. UICC monograph series, v. 4. [DNLM: 1. Neoplasms-Diagnosis. W1 U412 no. 4 / QZ241 I61c] RC270.I5 1974. 616.9'94'075. 74-18092

Offsetprinting and bookbinding Universitätsdruckerei H. Stürtz AG, Würzburg.

Foreword

The first edition of this Monograph on Cancer Detection was published by the International Union Against Cancer (U.I.C.C.) in 1966. Since that time the Committee responsible for that Monograph has gained considerable experience through the organization of a cervical screening programme in Santiago, Chile and a symposium on the evaluation of mass screening programmes in Sheffield, England. The knowledge acquired from these activities, together with the practical advice from participants and the introduction of new techniques of cancer detection have prompted the Committee to revise completely the 1966 publication. It is the hope of the International Union Against Cancer that this revision will prove helpful to all countries involved in or contemplating cancer detection programmes.

As the Chairman of the Cancer Control Commission within which the Committee on Cancer Prevention and Detection functions, I take pleasure in acknowledging their dedication and effort in the preparation of this report. The Committee members are:

* Dr. A. J. Phillips (Chairman) — Canada
  Dr. D. A. Boyes — Canada
  Dr. M. Gaitan-Yanguas — Colombia
* Dr. R. Gerard-Marchant — France
* Dr. J. Knowelden — England
  Dr. B. MacMahon — U.S.A.
  Dr. M. Montero — Chile
  Dr. T. Mork — Norway
  Dr. B. Terracini — Italy
* editorial committee

In the preparation of the report the Committee was assisted by Dr. John Wakefield, a member of the U.I.C.C. Committee on Public Education.

E. C. Easson M.D.
Chairman
Cancer Control Commission

Contents

Introduction

As was stated in the first edition, the overall purpose of this report is to guide those who are concerned with advancing the clinical control of cancer by increasing to a maximum the number of cases found at an early stage. In some respects the content may be considered as the standard for a cancer detection programme. However, the Committee responsible for its preparation recognises that factors which may be unique in some countries make it impossible to propose standards which would prove applicable to all countries. It is hoped, however, that the report will prove helpful to those who contemplate the first steps in a cancer detection programme and also to those who wish to expand programmes already in existence.

Cancer detection is based upon three assumptions, first, that treatment of benign and precancerous lesions reduces cancer morbidity, second, that treatment of *in situ* lesions reduces the cancer morbidity rate since such lesions frequently develop into true invasive carcinoma, and third, that early diagnosis and treatment of cancer means better therapeutic results. It should be pointed out that none of these assumptions has received complete clinical, statistical or experimental confirmation which has resulted in considerable diversity of opinion regarding the accomplishments and future promise of cancer detection activities. These doubts have been reinforced because for some sites of cancer, screening programmes have been followed by reductions in incidence rates but not by similar changes in mortality. Furthermore, uncertainty about the effect of a screening test is often based on too little knowledge about the natural history of the disease, for example in cancer of the cervix. Finally there is uncertainty about the best way of applying a screening procedure for maximum effect, whether to a total population or to a selected group most at risk. If the latter is adopted, there may be difficulties in defining this "at risk" group and practical problems of ensuring that these persons are adequately screened. Recognizing the need for careful study of the problems which have arisen in the field of cancer detection, the Committee on Cancer Prevention and Detection of the International Union Against Cancer (U.I.C.C.) convened a symposium to evaluate the effectiveness of mass screening techniques. The recommendations and decisions from this symposium have been interspersed throughout this report in appropriate places.

In addition to the symposium on evaluation of cancer screening programmes, the Committee has also had practical experience in the organization of a demonstration programme for cervical cytology screening. This activity emphasized many of the practical problems inherent in the development of cancer detection programmes and these have also been inserted in appropriate places throughout the text.

Since the education of the public plays such a prominent role in the organization of cancer detection programmes, a chapter on social and educational factors in cancer detection activities has been included. This was prepared by a member of the U.I.C.C. Public Education Committee, Dr. J. WAKEFIELD, and the Committee on Cancer Prevention and Detection wishes to express its appreciation for his contribution.

Chapter I

Biological Tests for Cancer

Whereas today the emphasis is on site specific tests for finding cancer early, there has been a long search for a general test which would shorten the period from the development of malignant cells to definitive treatment of the primary site. To some investigators, one of the most attractive of these was the Penn-Hall seroflocculation reaction for cancer supposedly produced when a bile-acid derivative was mixed with serum from cancer patients. However in 1957, PEACOCK and WILLIAMS reported the test unsuitable since it missed too many cancers and included too many false positives. Another test was for the appearance of lactic dehydrogenase isozymes (LDH) in human urine. WACKER and DORFMAN found elevated levels of LDH activity in the urines of 19 patients with known cancer but further clinical studies by RIGGENS and KISER showed that such elevations were not specific for malignant disease, and GELDERMAN attributed this to the presence of leukocytes or red cells in the urine.

The Shutz-Dale technique, a sensitive, immunological method as applied by MAKARI and corroberated by BURROWS, showed considerable promise but later investigators such as MAAS have been unable to confirm the original finding. Similarly, the Black-Kleiner-Bolker blood test suggesting that the plasmas of cancer patients gave very long reduction times for methylene blue, when subjected to critical analysis by ERIKSEN *et al.* proved insufficiently sensitive and not specific enough to differentiate cancer from other diseases. MENKES then introduced the possibility that serum from cancer patients displayed more sugar pentose than serum from normal individuals, but PEACOCK destroyed the idea by showing that there was doubt that serum destroyed pentose as a pentolysis phenomenon.

The Bolen test, developed in 1944, claimed that cancer could be diagnosed from "the blood pattern noted in a drop of blood on the glass slide", but upon evaluation by KASDON and HOMBERGER, it was discredited when the test was negative for many cancers in a group of cancer patients and positive in many normal patients. Then a test using the level of plasminogen in the serum of cancer patients was studied by PEACOCK and LIPPINCOTT, who reported no correlation between the plasminogen level and the nature of the disease.

The proposal that protein metabolism was abnormal in cancer patients was investigated by FISHMAN, BONNER and HOMBERGER by the determination of plasma glutamic levels but the results obtained in patients with and without cancer showed no difference.

More recently, immunologic diagnostic techniques have received attention, undoubtedly due to advancing immunologic technology and the increasing accumulation of information on immunological factors in oncogenesis. A number of these techniques appear to hold promise in the early diagnosis of human cancer. One of the first of these was the carcinoembryonic antigen (CEA) of the human digestive system first discovered by GOLD and FREEDMAN in 1965. Subsequently GOLD has described two different approaches to early diagnosis by immunological means, the first being to evaluate variations of immune reactivity which may accompany cancer growth and so determine whether a specific immunologic reaction has been evoked by certain specific tumour cell constituents.

In discussing this approach to immunologic diagnostic tests for cancer, GOLD writes as follows: "The hypothesis that tumour development may occur as a consequence of the breakdown of an immunologic surveillance mechanism has gained increasing prominence, if not universal acceptance. Support for this concept has come, for example, from the demonstration of an increased pre-disposition to cancer growth in patients with a variety of immunologic deficiency syndromes. For example, patients with various types of hypogammaglobulinemia appear to have an increased pre-disposition to the development of lymphocytic leukaemia. In addition, the family members of patients with chronic lymphocytic leukaemia manifest an increased incidence of hypogammaglobulinemia. Hence the study of the close relatives of patients with both immunoglubulin deficiency syndromes as well as lymphocytic leukaemia might prove quite fruitful in revealing a population-at-risk. The fact that individuals receiving immunosuppressive medication after organ transplantation have manifested a much higher incidence of *de novo* tumour formation than would be expected in a general population has added further credence to the relationship between tumour development and immunologic function. In the studies of the lymphomas where malignant cells have their origin in tissues intimately related to the immunologic apparatus, rather distinct patterns have emerged. Patients suffering from Hodgkin's disease most frequently demonstrate normal immunoglobulin levels and the ability to mount an adequate humoral immune response to primary and secondary stimulation with a variety of common antigenic materials. However, a state of energy, marked by a hiatus in cell-mediated immune responsiveness is found in $1/2$ to $2/3$ of such individuals when the disease has spread to multiple sites.

Individuals suffering from nonlymphomatous cancer also tend to develop defects associated primarily with cell-mediated immune responsiveness. In fact, it has been suggested that the preoperative capacity of the cancer bearing host to develop primary cell-mediated hypersensitivity to highly immunogenic haptens may correlate well with a favourable post-operative course of the disease.

Until recently it was believed that patients suffering from the leukaemias, lympho-sarcoma and reticulum cell sarcoma, unlike those affected with Hodgkin's disease or non-lymphomatous cancer, seldom manifest a significant degree of energy. It has been known for some time however that such individuals frequently develop either distinct elevations or depressions in serum immunoglobulin levels which, in either event, are associated with deficient humoral immune responses".

The second approach suggested by GOLD is the use of immunologic techniques in various assay procedures in order to detect the presence of characteristic tumour constituents in either the serum or secreted fluids of the tumour host. Such promise is placed in this approach that, at the present time, a number of immunoassay procedures are being developed for the detection of known tumourspecific or tumour associated constituents in the sera and other body fluids of cancer-bearing patients. In addition, GOLD points out that radioimmunoassays have in recent years become available for the quantitation of the circulating levels of a great many of the hormones e.g. the determinations for insulin, parathormone, thyrocalcitonin, ACTH, and a variety of the gonadotropins. Hence, radioimmunoassay techniques may be used for diagnostic purposes in endocrine tumours but identical technology has been employed in the investigation of non-endocrine tumours e.g. bronchogenic carcinoma.

To date a number of tests for circulating tumour-associated or tumour-specific antigens have been developed and tested. The more promising ones are:

a) Carcinoembryonic antigen (CEA) in the human digestive system. A radioimmunoassay has been developed which is capable of detecting quantities of the CEA, in nanograms, in the sera of patients with cancers of the bowel. In a number of instances the serologic diagnosis of cancer has preceded the demonstration of the tumour by conventional radiologic procedures. The test has been exposed to field trial in 5 university centres in Canada and the United States, which showed that it can be reproduced in other laboratories, albeit with some difficulty and without universal success, and that it is positive in a high proportion of patients with locally advanced colo-rectal cancer. The test has proved valuable in determining the prognosis in resected cases since a fall in the CEA level to undetectable concentrations suggests that the tumour has been entirely removed.

It is therefore of potential value as a diagnostic tool although its value as a screening procedure in asymptomatic patients remains to be assessed in large scale studies.

b) Alpha-Fetoprotein (AFP) in primary hepatomas. Reports originating from laboratories in different areas of the world have demonstrated the distinct value of a search for AFP in the sera of patients suspected of having primary hepatomas. The frequency with which the material reappears in the sera of such individuals varies from less than 50% to over 80% and shows marked geographic variations. In general it is higher in Afirca than in Western Europe. Field trials have shown this test to be an excellent diagnostic tool for primary liver cancer and is reproducable, highly specific, and fairly sensitive. It can be used for mass screening since it is possible to detect cases of primary liver cancer at the pre-symptomatic stage. However, even though the test meets many requirements for a good detection test, it has so far not been able to prevent the disease from following its fatal course.

c) Alpha H-Ferroprotein. This material is another protein that is normally present exclusively in human fetal organs and sera but is not normally found in the sera of children beyond the age of two months. Nevertheless, it has been detected in the sera of children suffering from teratomas and a variety of cancerous conditions involving the kidney, central nervous system and liver. In trial the test showed about 80% of the sera from such children gave positive results whereas only 8% of the sera from children with noncancerous diseases were positive.

d) Fetal Sulfoglycoprotein Antigen (FSA) in gastric cancer. Exploratory investigation has shown that this fetal type of Sulfoglycoprotein is found in the gastric juice of approximately 90% of patients with histologically proven gastric carcinomas. However about 10% of individuals without apparent gastric cancer also showed positive results. It is necessary therefore that a more sensitive technique for testing FSA is necessary.

e) Cancer Basic Protein (CaBP) in human neoplasms. This recent immuno-diagnostic test for cancer is based upon the principle that lymphocytes, sensitized to the protein, release a factor which inhibits the migration of marcrophages across an electric field. Lymphocytes from over 400 patients with proven cancer have given over 99% positive responses to the test while lymphocytes from "normal" individuals failed to release the macrophage slowing factor. The test appears to be highly sensitive but is essentially nonspecific since CaBP is present in all tumours.

This brief description of some of the work related to the diagnosis of human cancer which is being pursued by immunologically oriented investigators indicates that this discipline will undoubtedly make a substantial and practical contribution to the early detection of many malignancies.

Acknowledgement

Permission of the publisher Lea & Febiger, Philadelphia, to reproduce sections of "Immunologic Diagnostic Techniques— Phil Gold" from Holland&Frei *Cancer Medicine* is gratefully acknowledged.

References

BERGSTRAND, C.G., CZAR, B.: Demonstration of a new protein fraction in serum from the human fetus. Scand. J. clin. Lab. Invest., 8, 174 (1956).

BERSON, S.A., YALOW, R.S.: Radioimmunoassay of peptide hormones in plasma. New Engl. J. Med. 277, 640 (1967).

BOWER, B.F., GORDON, G.S.: Horomonal effects of nonendocrine tumors. Ann. Rev. Med. 16, 83 (1965).

BURROUGHS, D., NEILL, D.W.: Shultz-dale test for detection of specific antigen in sera of patients with carcinoma. Brit. med. J. 1958 I, No 5091, 368–370.

GATTI, R.A., GOOD, R.A.: Occurrence of malignancy in immunodeficiency diseases. A literature review. Cancer (Philad.) 28, 89 (1971).

GELDERMAN, A.H., BELBOIN, H.V.: Lactic dehydrogenase isozymes in urine from patients with malignancies in the urinary bladder. J. Lab clin. Med. 65, 163 (1965).

GOOD, R.A., FINSTAD, J.: Essential relationship between the lymphoid system, immunity, and malignancy. Nat. Cancer Inst. Monogr. 31, 41 (1969).

MAAS, H.: Der Immunologische Krebstest nach MAKARI. Klin. Wschr. 41, 120 (1963).

MAKARI, J.G.: The polysaccharide behavior of cancer antigens. Brit med. J. 1958 II, 5092 355 – 359.

National Cancer Inst. of Canada and the American Cancer Society. A collaborative study of a test for carcinoembryonic antigen (CEA). C.M.A.J. 107, July (1972).

OLD, L.J., BOYSE, E.A.: Immunology of experimental tumors. Amer. Rev. Med. 15, 167 (1964).

PEACOCK, A.C., WILLIAMS, G.Z.: A study of the Penn-Hall seroflocculation reaction for cancer. J. nat. Cancer Inst. 18, 277–283 (1957).

PENN, I., HAMMOND, W., BRETTSHNEIDER, L., SARZL, T.E.: Malignant lymphoma in transplantation patients. Transp. Proc. 1, 106 (1969).

PREHN, R.T.: Immunosurveillance, regeneration and oncogenesis. Progr. exp. Tumor Res. 14 (1971).

RIGGENS, R.S., KISER, W.S.: A study of lactic dehydrogenase in urine and serum of patients with urinary tract disease. J. Urol. (Baltimore) 90, 594–601 (1963).

SOUTHAM, C.M.: The immunologic status of patients with nonlymphomatous cancer. Cancer Res. 28, 1433 (1968).

THOMSON, D.M.P., KRUPEY, J., FREEDMAN, S.O., GOLD, P.: The radioimmunoassay of circulating carcinoembryonic antigen of the human digestive system. Proc. nat. Acad. Sci. (Wash.) 64, 161 (1969).

WACKER, W.E.C., DORFMAN, L.E.: Urinary lactic dehydrogenase activity. J. Amer. med. Ass. 181, 972 (1962).

Chapter II

Cancer Detection by Site

This chapter discusses those sites of cancer for which early detection techniques have been developed. The relative importance of each site in various countries is indicated in terms of its morbidity and mortality and the outcome of treatment is measured in terms of the five-year survival. Throughout the chapter it is to be understood that every lump and node, not obviously inflammatory, will be biopsied.

Buccal Cavity

Morbidity and Mortality

Cancer of the buccal cavity is not one of the most frequent cancers, nevertheless, it represents a serious problem when, in spite of its accessibility, diagnosis is made in the advanced stages of its evolution. Its frequency varies from one country to another and within the same country there are often areas with a higher incidence. The mortality data reported by Segi showing the variation between countries is shown in Table I.

Approximately 2% of all cancers are localized in the mouth (tongue, floor of the mouth, gums, cheek, soft and hard palate, anterior pillars and mucosa of the lip). The majority of these are squamous cell carcinomas. A few are adenocarcinomas arising from salivary glands and more rarely melanoblastomas. Sarcomas are exceptional.

Table I. Mortality rates by sex for cancer of the buccal cavity (SEGI, 1966–1967). Rate per 100,000

Male		Female	
Country	Rate	Country	Rate
France	10.0	N. Ireland	2.0
Switzerland	6.3	U.S.A. (non-white)	1.7
South Africa	6.1	Norway	1.6
Netherlands	1.5	Belgium	0.6
Israel	1.4	Japan	0.6
Japan	1.4	Germany (F.R.)	0.5

Prognosis

With the exception of the hard palate, each of the organs forming part of the mouth has a very rich lymphatic net, hence a very early transportation of tumour cells to the regional lymph nodes occurs, resulting in nodal metastasis. This explains why in approximately 5 to 10% of cases, the first manifestation of the disease is metastatic nodules in the neck. No doubt this is one of the reasons why present-day treatment results of 40% five-year survival are not as high as in some other equally accessible sites.

On the other hand, dissemination of the disease by the mechanism of direct invasion is very rapid and destructive in carcinoma of the oral cavity. This is especially true in the tongue and floor of the mouth. Distant metastases usually remain confined to the regional lymph nodes.

Two important aspects of carcinoma of the mouth are the frequency with which multiple lesions occur and the possibility of further, similar lesions of the upper respiratory or digestive tracts. This is not surprising since the entire mucosa in this region has presumably been exposed to the same carcinogenic agents and this should be kept in mind at follow-up examinations.

Detection Techniques

1. Clinical Examination

Direct examination of the mouth by inspection in good light and palpation are the most useful methods for detecting cancer of the buccal cavity. Unfortunately, they are not practised by doctors and dentists as frequently nor as thoroughly as they deserve. It is not the common procedure for a general practitioner to do a routine mouth examination in every patient. Even specialists in head and neck problems seldom do this for their interest is often limited to the eye, or the ear, or the nose. The same criticism can be directed to dentists; few of them making a complete examination of the entire buccal cavity. This problem is a serious one when one considers the malignant potentiality of many benign lesions, for example, leukoplakia, chronic ulcerations, etc. It becomes imperative, therefore, that special emphasis be directed to changes in former existing lesions. Another handicap is the fear of taking biopsies, in spite of the simplicity of this procedure. This, together with the previous considerations, explains why the diagnosis of oral cancer is often made at a late stage and why very advanced cases still present for treatment.

2. Exfoliative Cytology

The oral cavity, including the anterior aspect of the accessible oropharynx, is covered by squamous-cell mucosa, the total area being one of the largest in the body. On this basis alone, one might assume that exfoliative cytology should be a useful method of detecting cancer in this body cavity. Encouraged by the results obtained with the Papanicolaou method in early diagnosis of cervical carcinoma, many authors have conducted special studies on the application of this technique to the diagnosis of oral cancer. In spite of the many publications on the subject, not one study has been undertaken to detect cancer of the buccal cavity by cytological techniques in large groups of apparently healthy people. Some studies have been made of small groups but with special emphasis directed to the differentiation between benign premalignant conditions and cancer. Other studies have been directed to the follow-up of treated cases. Although there are still enthusiasts, the consensus of opinion in many large centres is that cytological diagnosis is unreliable for cancer in this site.

3. Biopsy

It is not necessary to insist on the simplicity of taking a biopsy, either by the general practitioner or by the dentist. However, it is worthwhile to insist that it must be obtained from the suspicious part of the lesion and in the case of leukoplakia it is advisable to excise the whole lesion and to make serial sections for study.

Stomach

Morbidity and Mortality

Stomach cancer is one of the most important diseases in respect to its relative frequency and actual mortality in many areas of the world. In Japan, for example, it accounts for over one half of all cancer deaths in men and over one third of all cancer deaths in women. Table II shows the mortality rates by sex for cancer of the stomach as reported by Segi.

Prognosis

Until etiological factors in gastric cancer are better understood and preventive measures can be applied, early detection and surgical extirpation are indispensable for best

Table II. Mortality rates by sex for cancer of the stomach
(SEGI, 1966–1967). Rate per 100,000

Male		Female	
Country	Rate	Country	Rate
Japan	66.8	Japan	34.6
Chile	56.5	Chile	34.2
Austria	40.0	Austria	22.5
Canada	16.4	Canada	7.6
Australia	15.6	U.S.A. (non-white)	7.6
U.S.A. (white)	8.5	U.S.A. (white)	4.4

control. Although cancer of the stomach is more common in men than in women, there is little difference in the overall survival picture. The five-year survival rate is approximately 12% but for patients with localized disease, the rate rises to 37% in men and 39% in women (End Results in Cancer, No. 4).

Symptoms in the early stage of stomach cancer are limited to mild anorexia, mild pain in the epigastrium, and mild fullness of the stomach. It is by no means infrequent that there are no symptoms whatsoever. As the disease advances the objective signs are: weight loss, increasing abdominal pain, occasionally anemia, and finally the so-called cachexia.

Detection Techniques

Four of many procedures helpful in the diagnosis of stomach cancer are:

1. Diagnostic procedures for gastric secretions.
2. X-ray examination.
3. Endoscopic diagnosis.
4. Cytological procedure.

Although each procedure brings about good results in the early detection of stomach cancer, a combination of these methods yields more exact early diagnosis. Consequently, it is usual to use two or more procedures in clinical practice.

1. Examination of Gastric Secretions and Scanning Procedures

Extensive studies of the stomach contents (gastric secretions), under fasting and stimulated conditions have indicated variations in acidity and enzymes in relation to benign and malignant disease but have not proved to be broadly useful for diagnostic purposes. Screening for low or absent acidity has been used as a means of identifying those individuals in the older, asymptomatic population who should be referred for further diagnostic examinations such as G.I. X-ray series, and can increase the yield of such procedures.

Techniques of scanning for early gastric cancer such as fluorescence (tetracycline) and radioisotope diagnosis using radioactive phosphorous (P_{32}) for selective pick-up, have been developed but have limited applicability.

As a general rule the early diagnosis of gastric cancer depends upon prompt application of radiologic and endoscopic procedures, with cytologic and histologic examination, in all groups and individuals where there is a clinical suspicion or group likelihood of this disease.

2. X-ray Examination

In advanced stomach cancer, X-ray findings are very obvious and diagnosis is easily made. However, in early stages the detection of the lesion by X-ray examination is by no means easy because the lesion is often limited to the mucus membrane and does not involve the entire thickness of the gastric wall. Roentgenographic changes in the gastric mucosa or gastric wall, at one time considered incidental, can now be identified as stomach cancer with the aid of gastric endoscopy. Since the introduction of the gastric endoscopic technique combined with the Roentgenographic examination, the early detection of stomach cancer has made great progress.

The first phase of the X-ray technique is designed for viewing the mucosa. A small amount of barium sulphate in suspension is swallowed in order to lightly coat the mucosa. To ensure even coating of all areas, outside pressure has to be applied (graded compression) to the area with some type of compressor (wooden paddle or other blunt instrument). Using this method, one can visualize irregularities of the mucosa. If any abnormalities are observed, a "spot film" should be taken with the patient assuming various positions, i.e. standing, supine, prone, the first oblique, and the second oblique.

To obtain an adequate "filling picture" of the stomach and proximal gastrointestinal tract, additional barium sulphate is administered. This mixture then fills the stomach and adjoining areas. The fluorescent screen or X-ray film will indicate any filling defects, i.e. rigidity, obstruction, constriction, etc. During fluoroscopy spot pictures can be taken of any abnormal areas. Again, the patient should assume the aforementioned positions when spot picture studies are required.

Mention should be made of the double-contrast method. After taking a sufficient amount of barium suspension, varying amounts of air are passed into the stomach through a tube. As a result the gastric wall is distended and outlined by a thin layer of barium. This method clarifies small elevations or shallow depressions in early carcinoma and also interruptions of the mucosal folds. This method in combination with the already mentioned "graded compression" and rotation of the position of the patient, is very effective.

3. Endoscopic Procedure

In 1956 HIRSCHOWITZ applied extra fine glass fibre to the gastroscope which is now called a fiberscope, and the pain to the patient was almost completely eliminated. This flexible instrument enables sufficient gross observation of the inner gastric surface and also colour photography of findings. This invention brought about a great advance in the early diagnosis of stomach cancer.

In Japan, for ten years prior to the invention of the fiberscope, the gastrocamera had been widely used. This consists of a thin flexible tube with a small camera at the tip. Photographs of the inner surface of the stomach can be taken in 32 consecutive shots on 8 mm colour film by the light from a lamp through the lens. These pictures are very sharp and realistically demonstrate even a minute change in the gastric mucosa. This method greatly enhanced the rate of detection of early stomach cancer. The shortcomings of the method are blind spot photography and difficulty in taking a picture of the cardia and fundus. The latter point was overcome by the invention of a retroflexible gastrocamera which takes pictures of the cardia and fundus. Now the gastrocamera is used routinely in Japan for detection of stomach cancer.

4. Cytologic Method

Observations made by roentgenography and endoscopy are only those of gross morphological changes. Confirmation of malignancy requires the study of histological or cytological observations to find the cancer cell itself. In this study the procurement and staining of intragastric cells are important. At present, there are the abrasive balloon method, the washing method, and the pressure washing method. Other methods such as washing with physiologic saline solution, papain solution, or kymotrypsin solution are also used. As for staining, there are Papanicoloau, May-Giemsa, aceto-gentian and fluorescence methods. Observation of fresh cells by the phasecontrast microscope is also a good method. It may be difficult to differentiate the cancer cells from noncancer cells in exfoliating cells. The gastric juice also has an effect on the cells, for which reason the differentiation may become more difficult. At this point, the most correct diagnosis is given by intragastric biopsy which is also useful for histological study.

For this purpose, a gastric biopsy resection of small pieces of the gastric lesion is performed under fiberscopic observation. At the Cancer Institute Hospital in Tokyo, intragastric biopsies are performed by means of small forceps attached to the top of the fibers-cope. It should be stressed that a combination of these methods brings about a greater degree of efficiency in the detection of early stomach cancer and increases the rate of detection.

Colon-Rectum

Morbidity and Mortality

The colon-rectum is one of the cancer sites accessible to direct examination and therefore presents an excellent opportunity for early detection and control. Here, early diagnosis is not only life-saving but can eliminate the need for extensive surgery and unpleasant prosthesis. Yet, even though several detection methods for early diagnosis of this disease are available, thousands of deaths from colon-rectum cancer occur annually in many countries.

The full extent of the problem of colon-rectum cancer has been clouded by the separate listing of the two sites statistically. Cancer registries publish incidence and mortality figures under such categories as "sigmoid", "rectosigmoid", "intestine", "large intestine", "colon", "rectum", and "large bowel". The colon and rectum are essentially one organ and should be listed as such. From the point of view of early diagnosis for cancer control and of premalignant polyp detection for cancer prevention, it is both logical and important that the distinction between colon and rectum be dropped and that the bowel below the ileocecal valve be considered as one organ. By combining the colon and rectum areas into one overall site, the major significance of findings in this site become clearly evident.

The contrasting national mortality rates for cancer of the colon-rectum most recently reported by SEGI, are presented in Table III. Every nation, race and social class is affected by this site of cancer which reflects multiple causal factors. Several studies on the causation of colon-rectum cancers are being conducted but the variables are many and complex and more time is needed before any new results are reported. Some of the established high-risk factors associated with this cancer are:

a) Adenomatous polyp and/or mucosal hyperplasia.

b) Familial polyposis.

c) Previous cancer of colon-rectum.

d) Ulcerative colitis.

e) Asbestos exposure.

f) Cigar smoking.

In a 1965 study from the Mayo Clinic, atypical cells were seen in 5.2% of adenomas with severe hyperplasia. As the condition approached anaplasia, or the *in-situ* phase, the changes became increasingly less distinguishable from one another. Thus, areas of mucosal hyperplasia in the bowel should be considered as precursors of polyps and excised when first observed or kept under periodic sigmoidoscopic observation. The mere presence of hyperplasia is an index of epithelial activity and indicates need for examination of the entire large bowel by barium

Table III. Mortality rates by sex for cancer of the colon-rectum (SEGI, 1966–1967). Rate per 100,000

Country	Male	Female	% of all cancer
Scotland	24.8	20.7	18.2
Denmark	22.9	19.2	15.7
Canada	21.5	19.0	18.1
Finland	10.8	9.1	14.9
Japan	8.3	7.1	7.5
Chile	5.9	6.8	8.7

enema X-ray studies. In cases of multiple areas of involvement, additional tests such as cytologic washings, should be considered.

The same Mayo Clinic study found that 64% of 1,000 diminutive polyps showed varying degrees of atypical changes. Over 50% of these polyps were 2 to 3 mm in diameter. On the other hand, the malignant potential of single polyps of the colon-rectum has been a widely disputed subject. ACKERMAN, SPRATT, and several others find no basis for the theory that adenomatous polyps do generate into carcinomas of the colon.

Although most adenomatous polyps and cancer of the colon and rectum occur in the sixth and seventh decade of life, every physician should be aware of the occasional occurrence of this disease in the young. BACON has compiled an excellent collection of cases of colon-rectum cancer in children.

Familial polyposis is a firmly established precancerous condition. Since it is known to be a genetically determined disease, all family members of a patient with polyposis should be examined and followed at regular intervals. Polyposis can involve a small area of the entire colon from the cecum to the anus. According to DAVID, the rectum is involved in 95% of the cases. An estimated 60% undergo carcinomatous change if this condition is not treated early. The most common sites of these growths, the sigmoid and the rectum, are within reach of a 25 cm proctosigmoidoscope, making early detection of all cases feasible.

The incidence of carcinoma of the colon-rectum in cases of chronic ulcerative colitis is close to 10% and presents an even greater danger to patients with long-standing, widespread involvement of the bowel. Ulcerative colitis over a period of 20 years gives a 40% increase in the incidence of colon-rectum cancer. One of the difficulties in detecting malignant change in this type of bowel is the already altered appearance of the mucosa. Since cancer superimposed on ulcerative colitis tends to be multicentric and undifferentiated, careful follow-up and re-examination of ulcerative colitis patients can prevent an unhappy discovery of advanced cancer at a later date.

Pseudopolyps develop in a large percentage of these cases, but are not the actual site of cancer development, cancer occurs in the surrounding, chronically inflamed and altered mucosa.

Although asbestos as a causative factor in lung cancer has now been firmly established, only recently have studies shown that there is a relationship between this substance and other neoplasms. SELIKOFF, CHURG, and HAMMOND as well as MANCUSO and COULTER have noted almost three times the expected rate of stomach and colon-rectum cancer in their study of U.S. asbestos workers. On the basis of these reports, asbestos exposure should be considered a predisposing factor but the degree of significance remains to be assessed.

It is now clear that smoking plays a significant role in the production of most cancers of the upper digestive tract but studies of U.S. veterans and British doctors do not show significantly different mortality ratios between smokers and non-smokers for cancer of the colon-rectum.

Prognosis

Although comparisons of results of treatment of cancer of the colon-rectum have been bedeviled by hostological criteria of malignancy—obviously the less invasive lesions result in better prognosis—the End Results Report indicates considerable improvement in the outcome of treatment over the past

Table IV. Five-year survival for cancer of the colon and rectum by stage—End Results no. 4, 1973

Stage	Five-year survival	
	Colon	Rectum
Localized	58%	50%
Regional extension	40%	24%

25 years. The results for the period 1955–1964 are shown in Table IV. Survival rates for women are consistently higher than for men and there is a constant decline in survival with age.

Detection Techniques

The following criteria for detection methods are not absolute but relative and many times interdependent. Nonetheless, they are good guidelines for evaluating cancer detection methods of the colon-rectum.

1. Physical Examination

Inspection of the perianal skin plus abdomen and nodebearing areas should precede the proctosigmoidoscopic examination. Any abnormality detected in this phase of the examination, even with a negative result from the proctosigmoidoscopic examination, should be investigated utilizing the barium enema.

2. Blood Tests

Hemoglobin and/or hematocrit determination as a routine part of an examination occasionally elicits a finding of unexplained anemia. In the absence of signs or symptoms pertinent to the bowel, there should be suspicion of a right-sided colon lesion and further

tests, including the barium enema, should be ordered.

3. Rectal Examination and Proctosigmoidoscopy

On the basis of figures compiled on autopsy and surgical specimens about 75% of all polyps and cancer arise in the rectum or rectosigmoid areas. Fig. 1 shows the proportion of cases detected by digital and sigmoidoscopic examination, indicating that 16% of carcinomas of the colon and rectum are theoretically within reach of the examining finger.

4. Guaiac Test

Occult blood in the stool or unexplained anemia often is the only clue to the presence of a lesion in the cecum or ascending colon. After a positive guaiac test, the next step in diagnosis is the barium X-ray examination.

5. X-ray Examination

Since approximately 20% of tumours of the colon-rectum are not within reach of the sigmoidoscope, the radiologist plays an important role in any complete study of this site of cancer. As mentioned previously, any clinical suspicion on history or physical examination requires "checking out" by barium enema.

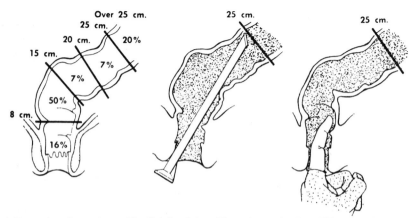

Fig. 1. Proportion of cases detected by digital and sigmoidoscopic examination (O'DONNELL, DAY, VENET)

Very small polypoid lesions are difficult if not impossible to detect by the conventional barium enema, hence air contrast techniques are an essential part of this detection method. Varying opinions on the percentage of accuracy of this technique exist, but this is due to the fact that the technique is only as good as the radiologist conducting the test. In the hands of a skilled radiologist the technique is highly accurate.

6. Cytologic Detection Technique

WISSEMAN et al. (1949) reported their results of applying the cytologic technique to 110 lesions of the colon and rectum. LATER, BADER, and PAPANICOLAOU (1952)

described their success with the technique in 200 colonic washings of patients.

Several methods of collecting cells have been used, some of which are the direct method where smears are made from material taken directly from visualized lesions; washings, where visualized lesions are washed with a saline solution which is then aspirated, preserved and studied; enema, where the enema results are strained, centrifuged and studied.

7. Biopsy

Obviously the final step in detection techniques is the biopsy, which allows for accurate identification.

Lung

Morbidity and Mortality

As a result of the rapid increase in recent years lung cancer is today one of the most common forms of cancer in many countries. It is still predominantly a disease among males, although significant increases in female rates are being reported. In all of the 24 countries surveyed by SEGI in 1966–1967 the age-adjusted death rates among females were lower than 10 per 100,000 per year and only 10 countries reported annual rates higher than 5. In contrast, the lung cancer death rates for males exceeded 20 per 100,000

Table V. Mortality rates by sex for cancer of the lung (SEGI, 1966–1967). Rate per 100,000

Country	Mortality rate	
	Male	Female
Scotland	78.1	11.7
England and Wales	70.0	10.7
Finland	61.0	3.9
Norway	14.9	3.0
Japan	14.0	4.9
Portugal	10.9	2.7

in 18 of these countries and were higher than 30 in 4 countries (see Table V).

Morbidity and mortality in this site of the disease both reach a peak among males in the age group 65–74 years. In 1966–1967 the death rate in this age group reached 600 per 100,000 in Scotland and exceeded 400 in several other countries in Europe.

These quoted figures refer to general populations. Very much higher mortality rates are observed among persons with a history of heavy cigarette smoking for 15 to 20 years or more. Compared with non-smokers, heavy cigarette smokers have at least a 20-fold risk of developing lung cancer. It is estimated that in countries with a high incidence of lung cancer such as Scotland, England and Wales, Finland, Austria, Belgium; at least 80% of all cases are ascribable to cigarette smoking.

In the causation of lung cancer today the magnitude of the effect of cigarette smoking far outweighs all other environmental factors. an occupational hazard is kown to exist among workers exposed to dust and fumes of radioactive material (as in uranium mines), nickel, chromate, beryllium, asbestos, various coal tar compounds, and possibly arsenic. However, nowhere is more than a very small fraction of the general population thus exposed.

Prognosis

Although there has been some improvement in the survival of lung cancer patients in recent years, the prognosis remains poor. Data from 5 countries show that in large series, including all diagnosed cases irrespective of stage and treatment, the 5 year relative survival rate is generally around 5–8%. These countries report much more favourable survival rates for localized cases treated by surgery—from to 25 to 30% 5year survival rate—but today less than 20% of all lung cancer cases belong to this fortunate category.

It follows from the foregoing that the key to effective control of lung cancer today should be *prevention* of the disease, by means of action directed at the known causative factors (cigarette smoking, occupational exposure). So far, however, attempts to achieve more than a transitory reduction of the cigarette consumption of the general population, have been strikingly unsuccessful. For the millions of persons who will be afflicted with this disease in the years to come, the only hope lies in earlier diagnosis and more effective methods of treatment.

Detection Techniques

The great majority of lung cancers develop from bronchial epithelium that has been exposed for years to tobacco smoke or the chemical compounds encountered in a limited number of occupations. Almost invariably this exposure results in demonstrable damage of the epithelium and underlying structures. The degree of damage depends on the duration of the exposure, the intensity of the exposure, the nature of the inhaled material, and on individual factors.

Common clinical manifestations of the damage are, "smokers cough", a feeling of shortness of breath, and demonstrable reduction of the breathing capacity. Among heavy cigarette smokers a substantial proportion gradually develops the syndrome of chronic bronchitis, with persistent productive cough, shortness of breath and more or less frequent episodes of acute inflammatory disease of the lower respiratory tract. The fact that respiratory symptoms such as these come to be regarded almost as "normal" among those most likely to develop lung cancer, is one of the main reasons for the present disastrous delay in the diagnosis of the majority of lung cancers. Any persistent symptoms from the lower respiratory tract in a person with a history of significant exposure, is a danger signal, and calls for adequate, periodic examination.

1. The Role of the General Practitioner

To establish the diagnosis of lung cancer usually requires the cooperation of a team of specialists. However, the specialists will not, as a rule, enter the scene unless and until they are called in by a general practitioner. Programmes for earlier diagnosis of lung cancer—as of cancer in general—must therefore give major attention to the general practitioner. Through his hands passes each year a large proportion of the adult population. It is he who is first consulted by the average person with early symptoms of respiratory disease. Among the large number of persons seeking him for a variety of other complaints, some will turn out to have symptoms from the respiratory organs in addition. In the flow of patients with and without respiratory symptoms, it is easy to identify those who are, on epidemiological grounds, classifiable as high risks with respect to lung cancer. As a general rule, irrespective of the reasons given for the consultation, those who belong to these high risk groups should be identified and then given adequate medical attention. Such a scheme would represent nothing new or unusual in patient-doctor relationship for the good doctor is always prepared to probe beyond the stated complaints of his patients and this is accepted and appreciated by the vast majority of them.

2. Guidelines for Early Detection of Lung Cancer

It is suggested that the following scheme be followed in areas where lung cancer presents a major problem. For reasons already given, the scheme is primarily recommended for use by general practitioners. However, it can and should be followed also by practising specialists, clinics, health centres and hospitals.

a) In persons over the age of 45 who come periodically for a general health examination, the scheme should include an annual X-ray examination of the chest. Fluoroscopy is not recommended for this purpose. The films must be read by a specialist.

b) As a routine, or whenever possible in connection with consultations, an attempt should be made to determine the exposure status of the individual in relation to lung cancer.

c) A chest film should be offered to all persons over the age of 45 who have been regular cigarette smokers for many years, and to all persons with a history of occupational exposure. This should be done even if respiratory symptoms are denied.

d) In the case of persons over the age of 45 who are heavy cigarette smokers (more than 20 cigarettes a day) or give a history of heavy occupational exposure, the time limit for periodic chest films should be reduced to every six months.

e) A chest film at six month intervals may likewise be recommended in the periodic control of exposed persons (smoking, occupation) with peristent symptoms from the lower respiratory tract even if the symptoms are considered no more than a "smokers cough".

f) Where facilities are available, the control of those who are heavy smokers or exposed to heavy occupational hazards should include cytologic examination of sputum. In general it has been found that if three or more samples are examined, a positive cytological diagnosis will be obtained in at least 80% of all lung cancers. The cytologic examination therefore is an extremely useful procedure in the search for early cases of this site of the disease.

To many readers the proposed scheme may seem drastic. Clearly, in many areas of the world, it is unnecessary and impossible today. However, in an increasing number of countries it is justified by the extremely high mortality from lung cancer in identifiable groups of the population.

3. Management of the Lung Cancer Suspect

If any of the examinations reveal abnormalities that may mean cancer, the question immediately arises whether the patient should be kept under observation by the general practitioner or placed in the hands of a specialist or a hospital. Whichever choice is made, the course of the disease should be closely watched with repeated chest films and it should be remembered that "atypical pneumonia", delayed resolution of a pneumonic infiltration, and recurrent pneumonia are very characteristic episodes in the development of lung cancer. They should be regarded as danger signs. In the follow-up of such episodes in high risk persons, repeated cytological examination of sputum samples is strongly recommended. Without exception, persons with abnormal or suspect cells in the sputum should immediately be referred to specialists or hospitals with all facilities for diagnosing lung cancer.

From this point it becomes an urgent matter to arrive at the correct diagnosis as quickly as possible. Unfortunately, very often considerable time is lost at this stage, even in technically advanced countries. GUISS found that while the majority of those found suspect on mass X-ray screenings sought medical aid, only 40% had a final diagnosis established in three months or less. Host, reporting on a similar survey found that for the lung cancer cases actually detected by the survey, on average, six months elapsed between the time of the survey and the time when the correct diagnosis was established.

It should be emphasized however, that those responsible for the management of the lung cancer suspect are often faced with extremely difficult tasks. It requires great knowledge and experience, technical skill and the ability to strike the proper balance between action and observation in each case. To obtain verification of the diagnosis, a prerequisite for instituting definitive treatment, is particularly difficult when the tumour is small and localized. Methods used in further pursuit of the diagnosis may include repeated chest film and cytological examination of sputum, special roentgenographic studies, bronchoscopy (if possible with biopsy), cytological examination of bronchial washings, scalene node biopsy, aspiration biopsy, pleural biopsy, and exploratory thoracotomy.

Breast

Morbidity and Mortality

According to SEGI (1966–1967) the age-adjusted death rate per 100,000 from cancer of the female breast ranged from 4.0 (Japan) to 26.5 (Netherlands) in the 24 countries covered by the survey. However, only four of these countries had death rates lower than 15 per 100,000 and fourteen had death rates higher than 20 (Table VI).

Table VI. Mortality rates for cancer of the breast (SEGI, 1966–1967). Rate per 100,000

Country	Mortality rate
Netherlands	26.5
Denmark	24.6
England and Wales	24.6
Portugal	11.9
Chile	9.7
Japan	4.0

In a large number of countries today, breast cancer is the most frequent form of malignant disease among women. In many urban areas the annual number of new cases exceeds 70 per 100,000 and in high risk groups, such as unmarried women over the age of 75, annual incidence rates as high as 400 per 100,000 have been reported.

Prognosis

The data reported by SEGI show that the mortality from breast cancer has remained relatively constant over the past 20 years and this has often been interpreted to imply that the survival experience of treated patients has also remained stable. However, according to the End Results in Cancer report the survival of 5 years for all stages of the disease has improved from 53% (1940–1949) to 63% (1960–1964). For localized cases, the improvement in the 5 year survival is shown to be from 78% to 84% and for cases with regional involvement from 42% to 53%. The 10 year survival rates for these two groups are 73% and 35% respectively. It is obvious that improvement in survival will result from an increase in the proportion of cases with localized disease.

Detection Techniques

With few exceptions, the first observation leading to diagnosis of breast cancer is made by the patient. The discovery of a lump in the breast, a sensation of heaviness or pain in the breast, observation of discharge from the nipple, scaling or excoriation of the nipple, or changes in the size or contour of the breast (retraction phenomena, dimpling) are the signs and symptoms which most commonly bring the patient to the doctor.

In many areas the patient will first be seen by a general practitioner. His examination will usually be confined to the classical inspection and palpation. Based on findings he will decide whether or not the patient needs to be referred to a specialist for further examination and treatment. It is therefore extremely important that general practitioners as well as specialists are thoroughly familiar with the technique of inspection and palpation of the breasts for abnormalities and that they have a clear understanding of when referral to specialists is indicated.

1. Inspection

Inspection should be carried out in good light and with the patient undressed to the waist. While the patient is sitting with her arms at her sides, the examiner will look for any evidence of disease such as lumps, asymmetry, or unilateral changes of the nipple (retraction, deviation, excoriation). It is essential that the two breasts be compared. Inspection should not be confined to the pendulous part of the breast, but should extend to the sternum and up to the supraclavicular fossa.

The patient is then asked to raise her arms above her head and as she does this, any changes in the contours of the breasts are noted. Inspection is extended to the axilla and the lateral part of the thoracic wall (see Fig. 2).

2. Palpation

Palpation should be carried out gently, with a relaxed hand, fingers together.

With the patient still in a sitting position the axilla is examined for evidence of enlarged nodes. One method of achieving the necessary muscular relaxation is to ask the patient to rest her left elbow in the doctor's left hand while his right hand explores her left axilla and vice-versa. Thereafter the supra and infraclavicular areas are carefully palpated (see Fig. 3).

The breasts are best palpated with the patient lying down. Palpation should be carried out first with the patient's arm at her side, then with the arm behind her head. In both positions the examination must be systematic, complete and careful so that no part of the breasts is overlooked. The examination must extend well beyond palpable glandular tissue, to the sternum, the clavicle, the lateral chest wall and below the inframammary ridge (see Fig. 4).

Normal breasts vary a great deal in size and consistency, being more or less firm, more or less glandular, lobular, scarred by previous mastitis etc. It is extremely important that general practitioners be familiar with this normal variation and this can best be achieved by making breast examination a routine in the examination of all female patients.

In this way only can the general practitioner—the key man because he usually sees the patient first—learn to react to those inconspicuous irregularities that *may* signal early cancer. Cancer detection at this stage is difficult but rewarding.

Whenever inspection and palpation bring to light any abnormalities, the physician has to decide whether referral to a specialist is needed. This is truly a critical stage in the examination of the patient. Although several considerations may enter into the decision, it will essentially be based on the interpretation of the results of the examination. This interpretation, however, is extremely difficult, particularly when lesions are small and it is precisely in these cases that it is of greatest importance to arrive at a correct diagnosis. The following data from a mass survey for breast cancer illustrate this point.

During this survey, general practitioners examined more than 70,000 women and they were encouraged to make unrestricted use of specialists. For each case referred to a specialist, the general practioners would state their interpretation of the findings at inspection and palpation. Table VII shows that among 111 cases classified by the general

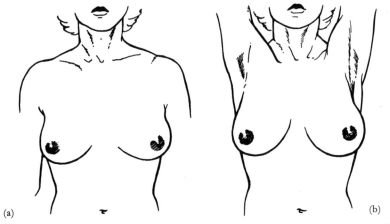

Fig. 2a and b. Inspection of the breasts with the patient sitting: (a) with the arms at the sides, (b) with the arms extended overhead[1]

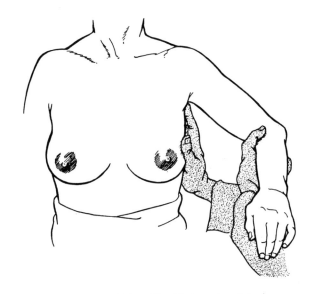

Fig. 3. Palpation of the axilla with the patient sitting[1]

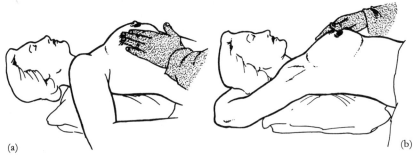

Fig. 4a and b. Palpation of the breasts with the patient lying down: (a) with the arms at the side, (b) with the arm behind the head[1]

---

[1] Figs. 2, 3 and 4 reproduced by kind permission of the C.V. Mosby Co., Saint Louis, Missouri, U.S.A.

Table VII. Variation in diagnosis of breast cancer

	Provisional diagnosis	Final diagnosis	
		Cancer	Benign
Suspect	111	17	94
Benign	629	23	606
Total	740	40	700

practitioners as suspect, 17 turned out to have cancer, while among 629 provisionally classified as benign, 23 actually had malignant disease.

3. Special Examinations

When a patient is referred to a specialist, his first step will be to repeat the classical inspection and palpation. Based on his interpretation of findings, he may proceed to a series of examinations aiming at an unequivocal diagnosis. These examinations require special skill and equipment and often necessitate hospitalization. They may include one or more of the following: cytologic examination of nipple discharge or fluid aspirated from cysts, soft tissue mammography, thermography, and biopsy. Among these mammography and thermography require special mention in that in some cases it is possible by these techniques to detect lesions too small to be found by palpation.

Biopsy with frozen section is the final step in the diagnosis of breast cancer. Incisional biopsy is generally considered superior to needle or trochar biopsy with frozen section. Definitive cancer therapy should never be started without microscopic confirmation of the diagnosis.

4. Breast Self-Examination

Since breast abnormalities are nearly always first noticed by the patient, it is a logical step to encourage all women to examine their breasts regularly and to teach them the technique of self-examination. Although this procedure has not been properly evaluated, it is a reasonable assumption that it may result in earlier detection of breast tumours. However, many women are unable to learn the technique properly from written material and doctors should take every opportunity to teach self-examination and to check that instructions have been correctly understood.

Female Genital Organs

Morbidity and Mortality

The U.I.C.C. Report on the Incidence of Cancer in Five Continents shows considerable variation in the relative frequency of cancers of the female genital organs (Table VIII). In addition, the mortality data provided by Segi show a similar variation and of approximately equal magnitude (Table IX).

The 15th Report on Gynaecological Cancer published by the "International Federation of Gynaecology and Obstetrics" (F.I.G.O.) gives information of some interest with reference to cancers of the female genital organs. The data submitted by 123 institutions from 26 countries for the period 1954–1963 show a ratio of 1:7 between cancers of the corpus and cervix (excluding carcinomas in-situ).

Prognosis

The F.I.G.O. Report presents the relative apparent recovery rates by stages for carcinoma of the cervix. These are as follows:

Stage 1 – 76.5%
Stage 2 – 55.0%
Stage 3 – 31.4%
Stage 4 – 8.8%

Table VIII. Age-Standardized incidence rates for cancer of the female genital organs. Five continents, UICC, 1970. Rate per 100,000

Country	Incidence rates		
	Cervix	Corpus	Ovary
Germany (DDR)	36.0	12.0	11.3
Puerto Rico	32.0	4.6	5.1
Denmark	30.8	11.0	13.5
Norway	16.2	8.2	11.5
Scotland	12.4	7.0	8.8
Israel (Jews)	4.9	8.8	11.4

Table IX. Mortality rates for cancer of the uterus (SEGI, 1966–1967). Rate per 100,000

Country	Mortality rate
U.S.A. (non-white)	22.2
Chile	20.1
Austria	17.7
Denmark	16.7
Norway	9.1
Israel	5.0

End Results in Cancer reports a 5 year survival of 79% for patients with localized disease and 45% for those with regional involvement. It is quite evident from these two reports which cover more than 130,000 cases of cancer of the cervix, that early detection is imperative.

Detection Techniques

For detection during the preclinical period of the disease, periodic medical examination must be perfomed including a pelvic examination. A thorough gynaecologic examination may include:

a) Clinical history of the patient.

b) Inspection of the external genitalia.

c) Visualization of the vagina and cervix with speculum.

d) Vaginal and cervical smears.

e) SCHILLER's iodine test.

f) Colposcopy.

g) Bimanual examination of the vaginal walls, cervix, fornices, uterus and adnexa. This will be completed with a combined recto-vaginal examination.

h) Endometrial aspiration, histerosalpingography and colpomicroscopy, when indicated.

i) Biopsy to confirm any diagnosis.

The patient's physician or the director of the detection programme, will decide upon the order to be followed according to the facilities at his disposal. If colposcopy is widely available it can play a part in screening, if not, exfoliative cytology can be a screening procedure with . colposcopy, Schiller's test and biopsy reserved for those cases with cytologic abnormalities. A brief description of these methods follows:

1. Exfoliative Cytology

For PAPANICOLAOU's cytology based on the spontaneous or induced exfoliation of the epithelial cells, there are numerous techniques to obtain material but what has gained wide acceptance is vaginal aspiration, cervical scraping, and endocervical aspiration or swabbing. Vaginal aspirates are obtained from the posterior fornix with a glass pipette; cervical smears by scraping around the external os (squamous columnar junction) with a cotton tipped applicator or a wooden spatula; endocervical aspirates with a thin metal canula, a glass pipette or a swab; and endometrical aspirates also with a thin malleable metal canula, a polyethilene tube with an attached syringe or a brush.

The following general rules should be followed:

a) Forbid douches, vaginal examination or sexual intercourse during the previous 24 hours.

b) Use dry pipette and canula, and unlubricated speculum.

c) Fix slides immediately.

d) Stain slides properly.

2. Schiller's Iodine Test

This test, based on the lack of glycogenic content of the abnormal epithelial cells, is not specific for cancer but useful to determine abnormal areas and to select the place where a specimen for a biopsy is to be taken.

3. Colposcopy

The colposcope, a binocular instrument, permits study under direct illumination of the vaginal and exocervical epithelia. Magnification of 10–40× is currently used. The cervical os is observed directly, after a gentle cleaning and after painting with a 3–5% aqueous solution of acetic acid for better transparency and with iodine for negative zones, to evaluate epithelial configuration, blood vessel arrangements, etc. Atypical changes, especially those of the squamous columnar junction lead to recognition of ectopy, transformation or transitional zones and areas of abnormal epithelia such as leukoplakia, grund, mosaic, iodine negative areas, vascular hypertrophy, abnormal trans-

formation zones, erosion vera and early carcinoma. In most cases colposcopy permits biopsy of the worst area on the cervix and therefore can lead to more precise management of early cervical neoplasia.

4. Biopsy

The examination of tissue obtained by biopsy is necessary for the definitive histologic diagnosis of malignancy. This may be a punch biopsy directed by colposcopy, multiple punch or wedge biopsies or cold knife conization of the cervix. Specimens should not be too small, torn, crushed or distorted and should be placed in a fixative solution and sent immediately to the laboratory with such pertinent information as patient's age, last menstrual period, recent treatments, clinical findings, tentative diagnosis and the exact source of the tissue.

The conization biopsy, in which a conical portion of the cervix is removed for serial section, becomes especially important when smears are positive and punch biopsies are negative. Electrocautery must not be used.

Male Genital Organs

Morbidity—Mortality—Prognosis— Detection Techniques

1. Penis

The incidence of carinoma of the penis shows considerable variation in the various countries of the world (SEGI) ranging from 3.2 per 100,000 males in Japan to 65.3 in non-whites in the U.S.A. In many countries therefore it can be classified as rare—often accounting for only 0.5% of all malignancies. Treatment results show approximately 60% of localized cases survive five years, while 25% of those with regional involvement survive the same length of time.

The diagnosis of carcinoma of the penis is obtained through physical examination followed by laboratory examination and biopsy.

In the physical examination, careful assessment of the cardiovascular system is necessary in view of the advanced age of many of the patients. In the laboratory examination blood uria estimation, WASSERMAN reaction and urine examination are done. In all cases of chronic lesions a routine biopsy must never be omitted. Only the microscopic examination can decide the nature of the disease.

The signs and symptoms of this site of the disease may be described as follows: cancers of the penis always begin as a small but definite lesion such as a wart, ulcer, sore, swelling or discharge often with a long history. More often, however, the foreskin cannot be retracted and the condition remains undiscovered until the tumour ulcerates. Attention to improved penal hygiene and circumcision soon after birth have been shown to be valuable preventive measures in this site of the disease.

2. Scrotum

Although cancer of the scrotum is relatively rare, approximately half as frequent as cancer of the penis, it's occurrence in pitch, tar and bitumen workers is recognized. Most of the tumours are ulcerating lesions. Some may be proliferative. All the early keratoses and papillary tumours are difficult to distinguish clinically from a malignant change. Pigmental lesions and melanoma are important considerations in this anatomical site. Histological examination of every lesion of the scrotum must be carried out.

3. Testis

Testicular tumours occur infrequently, the incidence rate per 100,000 ranging from 0.1 (Jamaica) to 4.5 (Denmark). The majority of testis tumours occur between the ages of 20 and 40 years, teratoma occurring most comonly between 20 and 30 years of age, and seminoma between the ages of 30 and 40 years. Early diagnosis is important in terms of outcome of treatment—the five year survival being 80% for localized cases and 60% for those with regional involvement. The best prognosis occurs in the seminoma.

The diagnosis of testicular tumours is made by inspection and palpation. The scrotum may show a unilateral enlargement, sometimes due to infection but most swellings are tumours. A minority may be gumma, infarcts, hematoceles, torsion of the spermatic cord and hydrocele. In palpation, the first point to be determined is whether the swelling is of the testis or epididymis. The most constant diagnostic characteristics of testicular tumours are hardness, heaviness and loss of sensitivity. Palpation should be exceedingly gentle because of the danger of disseminating metastases by handling.

4. Prostate

In many countries cancer of the prostate is the most common malignancy in men over the age of 65. However, the incidence and mortality rates vary considereably between countries. For example the mortality rate per 100,000 in Japan is 1.8 while in New Zealand it is 13.7. Treatment results show that approximately 65% of localized cases survive five years but only 46% of cases with regional involvement.

It is not difficult to obtain an accurate diagnosis of carcinoma of the prostate in patients with dysuria and retention of urine, when rectal examination reveals a large, hard and knotty asymmetric prostate. The early lesion may be difficult to differentiate clinically from benign conditions which also cause areas of induration.

The onset of prostatic carcinoma is frequently asymptomatic and occasionally may be detected during the investigation of other disease or on rectal palpation in the course of routine medical examination. Often the first symptom may be due to metastases. Approximately 15% of patients admitted to hospital suffering from urinary retention due to prostatic obstruction, will be found to have manifest prostatic cancer. It follows therefore that annual routine rectal examinations should be carried out in every male over 50 years of age. A malignant nodule is most commonly stoney hard, flat and not elevated above the surface of the gland and on palpation there is a marked difference in consistency between the nodule and adjacent tissue.

Bladder

Morbidity and Mortality

According to SEGI, the male mortality rate per 100,000 for cancer of the urinary system ranges from 7.9 in South Africa to 2.4 in Japan. Among females the rates are much lower, ranging from 2.7 among non-whites in the U.S.A. to 1.1 in Japan. Since most of the cases included under the heading of the urinary system will be cancers of the bladder, these statistics give a fairly accurate picture of this particular organ. In many countries the urological sites account for approximately 5% of all cancers—approximately 7% in males and 3% in females.

Prognosis

According to JAMES, the survival of Stage 1 cases at five years is 85.1%, Stage 2 is 40.8% and Stage 3 is 13.8%. Stage 4 has zero survival. In addition, the report End Results in Cancer shows a five year survival of 68% for localized cases and 18% for those with regional involvement. Fortunately approximately 75% of all patients are localized at diagnosis. Prognosis is poor among older patients and the overall survival rate of 68% for localized cases falls below 50% after 65 years of age.

Detection Techniques

In the diagnosis of cancer of the bladder, the following procedures are recommended:

a) *Physical examination*. Careful bimanual examination of the bladder is made under full surgical anaesthesis. Nearly the entire bladder is accessible to palpation by this method.

b) *Cystoscopy*. The identification of a tumour of the bladder is established usually by cystoscopy. Cystoscopic examination of all bladder tumours is essential. If blood is still recognisable in the urine cystoscopy should be carried out immediately.

c) *Laboratory examination*. If the bleeding has ceased, the urine should be investigated and cultured.

d) *Radiography*. Intravenous pyelography may reveal stones in the kidney, ureter, bladder, or prostate gland. The cystogram may show a filling defect caused by an intravesically projecting growth.

e) *Biopsy*. Endovesical biopsy which is not always possible, can be performed at the time of the cystoscopy. The tumour can be partly resected and the diagnosis established by microscopic examination. Biopsy is done whenever possible.

f) *Aspiration punction cytology*. In some centres, aspiration cytology is used for the exact identification of bladder tumours. This procedure requires a punction catheter which is generally a uretheral catheter having an injection needle fixed to one end. The material is aspirated by means of a syringe.

The early exact diagnosis of vesical lesions is very important because the possibility of any type of operative measure diminishes quickly with the progress of the disease. With the aid of such techniques as cystoscopy and intravenous or retrograde pyelography, a high percentage of urinary disorders can be accurately diagnosed today. In addition, exfolitative cytology now permits study of the malignant nature of a lesion while it is still very small making it possible at times to discover carcinomas of the urinary tract that are still in the early even pre-invasive developmental phase.

Routine cytological screening of the urine has been widely used in high risk industrial populations where, for example, the excretion of carcinogens is common. In the dye industry, where aniline dyes are associated with bladder cander, the workers must be examined annually with routine cytological screening. Such a procedure could also be done for patients with bilharziasis in whom cancer of the bladder may develop.

The symptoms of cancer of the bladder are haematuria, dysuria, pain, and tumour. The most common symptom in the case of vesical tumours is haematuria. This is usually painless in about three quarters of the patients. It may be profuse or slight, transient or persistent, early or late and may occur with obstruction. Haematuria requires complete physical and urological investigation.

Skin

Morbidity and Mortality

Cancer of the skin is one of the more common types of malignant disease and in some countries accounts for as much as 20% of all cancers. As a general rule it is more frequent in areas where there is a high exposure to the sun or where the light intensity is high because of the perpendicular path of the sun's rays, or lastly because of altitude.

Table X shows the variation in the incidence of cancer of the skin in various countries.

The skin has the peculiarity that it can be affected by different histological types of cancer, each with its own special type of behaviour. For example, basal-cell carcinoma represents about 80% of all skin cancers which fortunately very seldom give rise to metastasis; squamous cell carcinoma of the skin, on the other hand, accounts for about 15% of all cases and is certainly malignant. Finally, melanoblastoma, one of the most agressive tumours in the body, accounts for about 5% of all skin cancers.

Detection Techniques

There is probably no other organ in the body where clinical examination is as important and as exclusive for the diagnosis of cancer as it is in the skin. A careful clinical inspection and palpation can discover almost 100% of skin cancers. All lesions should of course be biopsied in order to confirm or clarify clinical findings. In general, the biopsy is a simple procedure even in the office of a general practitioner and it is recommended that the complete lesion be excised for histological study if the location and size permit. Special attention and biopsy procedures however, should be given to pigmented skin tumours. In these cases incisional biopsy should be avoided since it may cause dissemination of the malignant cells.

Table X. Age-Standardized incidence rates for cancer of the skin. Five continents, UICC, 1970. Rate per 100,000

U.S.A. (Texas)	169.2
South Africa	133.0
Canada	53.0
Hungary	30.3
Japan	1.5
India	1.3

Thyroid Gland

Morbidity and Mortality

Cancer of the thyroid gland accounts for approximately 1.0% of all cancer mortality. On the other hand, the incidence of thyroid cancer is much higher as these tumours are curable in a high proportion of cases.

Schematically there are 4 anatomo-clinical types with different etiological, clinical and course characteristics (Table XI).

Table XI. Summary of cancers of the thyroid gland

Type	%[a]	Age	Tumour	Lymph node metastasis	Distant metastasis	Prognosis
Papillary	70	peak: 3rd decade, children adolescent	small sometimes occult	very frequent, sometimes "primary"	uncommon	generally good (patient may survive a long time with cancer)
Follicular	15	peak: 4th decade	nodule	uncommon	frequent, sometimes "primary" (bones, lungs)	may be good (metastases controlled by I^{131})
Anaplastic	10	peak: after the 5th decade	fulminating growth with obstructive troubles	frequent, makes a single mass with the thyroid tumour	uncommon (death occurs before metastasis)	very poor
Medullary	5	peak: 4th decade	nodules	very frequent	late (bone, liver)	fair (patient may survive a long time with cancer)

[a] Percentages differ slightly from country to country.

Many factors are often involved in the etiology of thyroid carcinoma, such as geographic location, primary nodular goiter (adenoma), neck and mediastinum X-ray therapy in childhood, whole body irradiation and genetic for medullary carcinoma.

Geographic location is demonstrated by mortality statistics (Table XII). The highest mortality rates are observed in mountain areas and areas far from the sea and consequently with a lack of iodine in the diet. The frequencies of iodine deficiency, endemic goiter and thyroid cancer tend to parallel eachother.

Table XII. Relationship of geographic location and mortality for cancer of the thyroid gland (SEGI, 1966–1967)

Country	Death rate per 100,000	
	Male	Female
New Zealand	0.49	0.60
Belgium	0.52	0.66
Austria	1.15	1.54
Switzerland	1.16	1.34

Primary nodular goiter has been and is the subject of great debate as far as its relationship to carcinoma is concerned. But the question is not the possible influence of an adenomatous nodule on the etiology of thyroid carcinoma, it is the problem of clinical diagnosis between benign and malignant nodules.

The effect of X-ray therapy on the neck and upper mediastinum was demonstrated by CLARK. The incidence of thyroid cancer appears highest in patients who received radiation when children.

Whole-body irradiation appears to increase the incidence of thyroid carcinoma as demonstrated by studies on Japanese exposed to the atom bomb (ANGEVINE and JABLON).

Medullary carcinoma, a tumour developed from the parafollicular (C) cells can be a familial disease and is sometimes associated with other endocrin tumours such as pheochromocytoma.

Detection Techniques

In some instances, the first evidence of thyroid carcinoma is a cervical lymph node metastasis or a distant metastasis. The histological examination of the biopsies will point to the thyroid gland.

For the medullary carcinomas, the first symptoms are often functional (diarrhea). The level of thyrocalcitonin in the blood permits recognition of the type of cancer before the histological analysis. In most cases, however, the problem relates to a thyroid nodule. Isotopic study should be the first step. Since thyroid carcinomas are almost never functional, a concentrating (hot) nodule is schematically never carcinomatous, while a non-concentrating (cold) nodule is very suspicious—15 to 30% of them being malignant.

In the case of the hot nodule, a careful and regular follow-up of the patient is recommended. In the case of a cold nodule however, a few techniques have been proposed to rule out or assess the malignancy. Clinical examination should look for any suspicious lymph node in the neck. Laryngeal study must be systemic but has almost no value in the early diagnosis as vocal cord palsy generally indicating a recurrent laryngeal nerve involvement is only observed in advanced, extracapsular carcinomas. Radiographic study of the thyroid using special techniques for soft tissue will search for a psammoma which is always associated with papillary carcinoma. Punction biopsy has a direct interest—to empty a cyst which is a frequent lesion and is cold on scintigram. However, the pathological value of punction biopsy or drill biopsy is limited and BOEHME demonstrated that histological diagnosis on punction biopsy was accurate in only 57% of cases. Moreover Punction biopsy has risks. It may induce haemorrhagic necrosis in a nodule and hematocele, or it may induce grafting of tumour cells in soft tissues. If punction demonstrates a cyst, it does not indicate its nature, that is, a common cyst or a papillary cystadenocarcinoma.

Therefore, surgical exploration of the neck is often the last step of these studies and allows examination of nodule or lymph nodes which, after frozen sections, give immediate therapeutic conclusions.

Careful pathological study also provides a step in detection. Every thyroid surgically removed, whatever the clinical diagnosis, must be microscopically analysed with great care and *in toto*. This need clearly appears in Table XIII after LINDSAY.

Table XIII. Diagnosis of thyroid carcinomas, first established clinically, at operation or in the pathological laboratory

	Clinical	Surgical	Patho-logical	Total
Papillary	66	32	76	174
Follicular	29	11	43	83
Anaplastic	23	2	0	25

References

Buccal Cavity

ANDERSON, D.L.: Cause and prevention of lip cancer. J. Canad. dent. Ass. **37** (4), 138–142 (1971).

ARSENAULT, J.M.: Cytology and its role in the detection of oral cancer. Cancer Cyt. **5** (1), 33–38 (1964).

AYRE, W.B.: The manifestation of disease as revealed by oral cytology. Cancer Cyt. **4** (1), 4–14 (1961).

HOPP, E.S.: Cytologic diagnosis and prognosis in carcinoma of the mouth, pharynx and nasopharynx. Laryngoscope (St. Louis) **68**, 1281–1287 (1958).

HOROWITZ, R., CHOMET, B.: Oral carcinoma and multiplidity of carcinomas. Oral Surg. **26**, (1), 87–91 (1968).

KING, O.: Oral cytology for the general practitioner. Amer. dent. Ass. **66**, 451–455 (1963).

KING, O., COLEMAN, S.: Analysis of oral exfoliative cytologic accuracy by control biopsy technique. Acta cytol. **9** (5), 351–354 (1965).

PAPANICOLAOU, G.N.: Atlas of exfoliative cytology. Cambridge: Harvard University Press 1954.

PETERS, H.: Cytologic smears from the mouth; cellular changes in disease and after radiation. Amer. J. clin. Path. **29**, 219–225 (1958).

SANDLER, H.: The detection of early cancer of the mouth by exfoliative cytology. Acta cytol. **5** (3), 191–194 (1961).

SANDLER, H.: Oral exfoliative cytology for detection of early mouth cancer. Acta cytol. **6** (4), 355–358 (1962).

SILVERMAN, S., JR. et al.: al.: The diagnostic value of intraoral cytology. J. dent. Res. **37**, 192–205 (1958).

UMIKER, W.O.: The grading of squamous cell carcinoma by cytologic smears; a preliminary report. Univ. Mich. med. Bull. **23**, 353–355 (1957).

UMIKER, W.O.: Oral and laringeal exfoliative cytology. Cancer Cyt. **5** (1), 27–32 (1964).

Stomach

CHIDA, N., et al.: Cytology of early stomach cancer. Diagnostic limitation. Jap. J. Clin. **23**, 495–508, 711–725 (1965).

HAFTER, E.: Praktische Gastroenterologie. Stuttgart: Georg Thieme 1962.

ICHIKAWA, H.: X-ray diagnosis of early stomach cancer. J. Clin. digest. Dis. (Tokyo) **5**, 557–567 (1963).

ICHIKAWA, H.: X-ray diagnosis of early gastric cancer. Recent progress of diagnosis technique. Jap. J. Cancer Clin. **9**, 683–692 (1963).

ICHIKAWA, H.: X-ray diagnosis of the stomach. Tokyo: Kobundo 1964.

ICHIKAWA, H.: X-ray diagnosis of early stomach cancer. Clin. All-Round (Tokyo) **14**, 1657–1666 (1965).

KAJITANI, T., et al.: Early stomach cancer. Jap. J. intern. Med. **16**, 212–216 (1965).

KEMEYA, S., et al.: A new-type gastro-fiberscope equipped with a glassfiber light guide. Gastroent. Endoscopy (Tokyo) **6**, 36–40 (1964).

KAWAMATA, K., et al.: Clinical aspects of early stomach cancer. Surg. Tber. (Tokyo) **13**, 263–274 (1965).

KIDOKORO, T., et al.: Gastrocamera and cytology of early stomach cancer. Surg. Ther. (Tokyo) **10**, 45–52 (1964).

KIDOKORO, T., et al.: Endoscopic diagnosis of early stomach cancer. Jap. J. Clin. (Kyoto) **22**, 1871–1877 (1964).

KOSAKI, G., et al.: Diagnosis of early stomach cancer. Surg. Ther. (Tokyo) **13**, 37–52 (1965).

KUROKAWA, T.: Early detection of stomach cancer. Acta Un. int. Cancr. **18**, 760–765 (1962).

MASSA, J.: Le petit cancer de la stomach. Paris: Masson & Cie. 1961.

MASUDA, M., et al.: Endoscopic studies of early stomach cancer. J. Clin. dig. Dis. (Tokyo) **6**, 963–972 (1964).

MIYAJIMA, S., et al.: Early stomach cancer detected by gastric mass survey. J. Clin. dig. Dis. (Tokyo) **6**, 1376–1384 (1964).

MORIWAKI, H., et al.: X-ray diagnosis of early stomach cancer. Silhouette findings. Clin. Radiol. (Tokyo) **10**, 465–475 (1965).

MURAKAMI, T.: Early gastric cancer. Gann Monograph on Cancer Research II, Japanese Cancer Ass. Tokyo, 1971.

OKUDA, S.: Diagnostic limitation of endoscopy of early stomach cancer. Jap. J. Clin. (Kyoto) **23**, 481–494, 700–710 (1965).

PANEL Discussion of IV Congr. of Japan Endoscopy Society, Early Stomach Cancer. Gastroent. Endoscopy (Tokyo) **4**, 130–201 (1962).

SAKITA, T., et al.: Gastrocamera diagnosis of early stomach cancer. J. Clin. dig. Dis. (Tokyo) **5**, 746–749 (1963).

SASAKI, T.: X-ray examination of early stomach cancer. Clin. Radiol. (Tokyo) **9**, 520–531 (1964).

SEINO, S., et al.: X-ray findings of superficial early stomach cancer. Clin. Radiol. (Tokyo) **10**, 476–485 (1965).

SHIDA, S., et al.: Cytology of early stomach cancer. J. Clin. dig. Dis. (Tokyo) **5**, 711–763 (1963).

SHIRAKABE, H., et al.: X-ray diagnosis of early stomach cancer. Surg. Ther. (Tokyo) **10**, 31–44 (1964).

SHIRAKABE, H., et al.: Recent progress of diagnosis of early stomach cancer. Jap. J. intern. Med. **14**, 227–2355 (1964).

Symposium of II Autamnal Congr. of Japan Endoscopy Society, 1965 Diagnosis of superficial early stomach cancer, vol. 6, p. 323–345.

Symposium of VI Congr. of Japan Endoscopy Society & III Congr. of Japanese Society of Gastric Mass Survey. Cytology of early stomach cancer. Gastroent. Endoscopy (Tokyo) **6**, 110–124 (1964)—Gastric Cancer (Tokyo) **4**, 95–119 (1964).

Symposium of VI Congr. of Japan Endoscopy Society & III Congr. of Japanese Society of Gastric Mass Survey: Early stomach cancer detected by stomach mass survey. Gastroent. Endoscopy (Tokyo) **6**, 84–109 (1964);—Gastric Cancer (Tokyo) **4**, 4–58 (1964).

TAKEMOTO, T., *et al.*: Diagnosis of early stomach cancer. Significance of endoscopic observation. J. Clin. dig. Dis. (Tokyo) **5**, 750–762 (1963).

TASAKA, S.: Statistics of early stomach cancer in Japan, Gastroent. Endoscopy **4**, 4–14 (1962).

TSUJI, S.: Clinical studies of polypoid lesions and early stomach cancer. J. Kyoto Prefect. med. Univ. **72**, 748–749 (1963).

TSUNEOKA, K., *et al.*: Fibergastroscopic diagnosis of early stomach cancer. Jap. J. intern. Med. **14**, 237–245 (1964).

WATANUKI, S., *et al.*: Gastrocamera and cytology of early stomach cancer. J. Clin. dig. Dis. (Tokyo) **6**, 812–819 (1964).

YAMADA, T., *et al.*: Cytology of early stomach cancer. Kymotrypsin washing. J. Clin. dig. Dis. (Tokyo) **5**, 772–780 (1963).

YAMAGATA, S.: Clinical aspects of the early cancer of the stomach. Jap. J. Cancer Clin. **11**, 493–499 (1965).

YAMAGATA, S.: Clinical studies of early stomach cancer. X-ray diagnosis. J. Clin. dig. Dis. (Tokyo) **6**, 599–608, 691–707, 802–811, 984–990 (1964).

YAMAGATA, S.: Significance of cytology and biopsy for diagnosis of early stomach cancer. Jap. J. Clin. (Kyoto) **22**, 1878–1892 (1964).

YAMAGATA, S.: Cytology of stomach cancer with fiber-gastroscopic washing equipment (fibergastroscope K-type). III Autumnal Congr. of Japan Endoscopy Society, Sapporo 1965.

YOKOYAMA, H., *et al.*: Diagnostic evaluation of fiberscope. J. Clin. dig. Dis. (Tokyo) **5**, 789–798 (1963).

Colon-Rectum

ACKERMAN, L.V.: Is it cancer? Will it become cancer? proc. Fourth Nat. Cancer Conf. Minneapolis, 1960, p. 97–112. Philadelphia: J.B. Lippincott Co. 1961.

ACKERMAN, L.V., KRAUS, F.T.: The pathology of tumors. I. Introduction, precancerous lesions, and benign lesions that resemble cancer. Cancer (Philad.) **12**, 222–232 (1962).

ALLCOCK, J.M.: An assessment of the accuracy of the clinical and radiological diagnosis of carcinoma of the colon. Brit. J. Radiol. **31**, 272 (1958).

American Cancer Society, 1974. Cancer Facts and Figures. New York: American Cancer Society, Inc. 1964.

ANDREN, L., FRIEBERG, S.: Frequency of polyps of rectum and colon, according to age, and relation to cancer. Gastroenterology **36**, 631 (1959).

ANTHONISEN, P., RIIS, P.: Cytology of colonic secretion in proctosigmoidal disease. Acta med. scand. **172**, 375–381 (1962).

BADER, G.M., PAPANICOLAOU, G.N.: The application of cytology in the application of cytology in the diagnosis of cancer of the rectum, sigmoid and descending colon. Cancer (Philad.) **5**, 307–314 (1952).

BARGEN, J.A.: The nature of carcinoma associated with ulcerative colitis. Dis. Colon Rect. **5**, 356–360 (1962).

BROOKE, B.N.: Malignant change in ulcerative colitis. Dis. Colon Rect. **4**, 393–398 (1961).

BURN, J.I.: Exfoliative cytology of the colon. Proc. roy. Soc. Med. **54**, 726–729 (1961).

BURN, J.I. SELLWOOD, R.A.: The results of exfoliative cytology studies in 50 patients with symptoms of large bowel disorder. Gut **3**, 32–37 (1962).

CAMERON, A.B., THABET, R.J.: Recovery of malignant cells from enema returns in carcinoma of the colon. Surg. Forum **10**, 30–33 (1959).

CAMERON, A.B., THABET, R.J.: Sigmoidoscopy as part of routine cancer clinic examinations with correlated fecal chemistry and colon cytologic studies Surgery **48**, 344–350 (1960).

CASTLEMAN, B., KRICKSTEIN, H.I.: Do adenomatous polyps of the colon become malignant? New Eng. J. Med. **267**, 469–475 (1962).

COOK, G.B.: Silicone-foam enema as a diagnostic aid in cancer of the rectum and colon. Dis. Colon Rect. **7**, 195–196 (1964).

COOLEY, R.N., AGNEW, C.H., RIOS, G.: Diagnostic accuracy of the barium enema study in carcinoma of the colon and rectum. Amer. J. Roentgenol. **84**, 316 (1960).

DAY, E.: Value of simple procedures in cancer examinations. In: Cancer (RONALD RAVEN, ed.), vol. 3, p. 445. London: Butterworth & Co. 1958.

DAY, E.: Detection of cancer of the colon and rectum. Acta Un. int. Cancr. **18**, 766–771 (1962).

DAY, E.: Fourth Nat. Cancer Conf., p. 705–707. Philadelphia: J.B. Lippincott Co. 1961.

DUKES, C.E.: Simple tumors of the large intestine and their relation to cancer. Brit. J. Surg. **13**, 721 (1925).

DUKES, C.E.: The hereditary factor in polyposis intestini or multiple adenomata. Cancer Rev. **5**, 241 (1930).

DUKES, C.E.: The control of precancerous conditions of the colon and rectum. Canad. med. Ass. J. **90**, 630–635 (1964).

EDWARDS, C.C., JACKMAN, R.J.: Unsuspected and subclinical lesions of the large intestine found at necropsy. Surg. Gynec. Obstet. **105**, 754 (1957).

ESSER, J.G. VAN: The cytologic detection of cancer of the colon. Ned. T. Geneesk. **105**, 1849–1851 (1961).

GALAMBOS, J.T.: Cytologic examination of benign colonic lesions. Acta cytol. (Philad.) **6**, 148–154 (1962).

GILBERTSEN, V.A.: Adenocarcinoma of the large bowel: 1,340 cases with 100 per cent follow-up. Surgey **46**, 1027 (1959).

HAENSZEL, W., CORREA, P.: Cancer of the colon and rectum and adenomatous Polyps. Cancer (Philad.) **28** (1), 14–24 (1971).

HEIDENREICH, A.: Rectocolic exfoliative cytology. Pren. méd. argent. **47**, 2009–2019 (1961).

HENNIG, N., WITTE, S.: Atlas der gastroenterologischen Cytodiagnostik. Stuttgart: Georg Thieme 1957.

HERTZ, R.E.L., DEDDISH, M.R., DAY, E.: value of periodic examinations in detecting cancer of the rectum and colon. Postgrad. Med. **27**, 290–294 (1960).

JAMES, A.G.: Cancer prognosis manual. Amer. Cancer Society, Inc. 1961.

MANCUSO, T.F., COULTER, E.J.: Methodology in industrial health studies. Arch. industr. Hyg. **6**, 210–226 (1963).

MORSON, B.C.: Precancerous lesions of the colon and rectum. J. Amer. med. Ass. **179**, 316–321 (1962).

OAKLAND, D.J.: New way of diagnosis of carcinoma of the large bowel. Brit. J. clin. Pract. **16**, 707–715 (1962).

O'DONNELL. W.E., DAY, E., VENET, L.: Early detection and diagnosis of cancer. St. Louis: C.V. Mosby Co. 1962.

PAGTALUNAN, R.J.G., DOCKERTY, M.B., JACKMAN, R.J., ANDERSON, M.J.: The histopathology of diminutive polyps of the large intestine. Surg. Gynec. Obstet. **120**, 1259–1265 (1965).

PAPANICOLAOU, G.N.: Atlas of exfoliative cytology. Cambridge: Harvard University Press 1954.

PINI, C.E., BRACCINI, C.: Experimental, histological and clinical considerations on the concept of precancerous lesions. Panminerva med. **4**, 428–434 (1962).

RASKIN, H.F., KIRSNER, J.B., PALMER, W.L.: Exfoliative cytology of the gastrointestinal tract. In: Modern trends in gastroenterology (F.A. JONES, ed.) (2nd Ser.). London: Butterworth & Co. 1958.

RIDER, J.A., KIRSNER, J.B., MOELLER, H.C., PALMER, W.L.: polyps of the colon and rectum: A four-year to mine-year follow-up study of five hundred thirty-seven patients. J. Amer. med. Ass. **170**, 633 (1959).

RIIS, P., ANTHONISEN, P.: A new method of proctological diagnosis based upon cytological principles. Ugeskr. Laeg. **123**, 1713–1721 (1961).

RIJSSEL, T.G. VAN: The development of malignancy from precancerous lesions. Acta Un. int. Cancr. **12**, 718–722 (1956).

ROTH, S.I., HELWIG, E.J.: Juvenile polyps of th rectum and colon. Cancer (Philad.) **16**, 468–479 (1963).

SELIKOFF, I.J., CHURG, J., HAMMOND, E.C.: Asbestos exposure and neoplasia. J. Amer. med. Ass. **188**, 22–26 (1964).

SLANEY, G., BROOKE, B.N.: Cancer in ulcerative colitis. Lancet **1959 II**, 694.

SPJUT, H.J., MARGULIS, A.R., COOK, G.G.: The silicone-foam enema: A source for exfoliative cytological specimens. Acta cytol. (Philad.) **7**, 78–84 (1963).

SPRATT, J.S., JR., ACKERMAN, L.V., MOYER, C.A.: Relationship of polyps of the colon to colonic cancer. Ann. Surg. **148**, 682 (1958).

STEWART, F.W.: The problem of the precancerous lesion. Postgrad. Med. **27**, 317–323 (1960).

Lung

DUGUID, H.L., HUISH, D.W.: Clinical evaluation of the in bronchial carcinoma. Brit. med. J. **1963** , No 5352, 287–291.

Health consequences of smoking. Report of the Surgeon General-1972, U.S. Dept. of Health, Education & Welfare.

HOST, H.: The value of periodic mass chest roentgenographic survey in the detection of primary bronchial carcinoma in Norway. Cancer (Philad.) **13**, 1167–1184 (1960).

LILIENFELD, A.: ACS-Va Cooperative study for evaluation of radiologic and cytologic screening in the early detection of lung cancer. Acta Un. int. Cancr. **19**, 1130–1334 (1963).

O'DONNELL, W.E., DAY, E., VENET, L.: Early detection and diagnosis of cancer, 286 p. St. Louis: C.V. Mosby Co 1962.

Second world conference on smoking and health. Pitman House, Parker St., London, 1972.

SEGI et al.: Cancer mortality for selected sites in 24 countries. Department of Public Health, Tohoku University School of Medicine, Sendai, Japan 1964.

Smoking and health. Report of the Advisory Committe to the Surgeon General of the US Public Health Service. Public Health Service Publication No 1103. US Government Printing Office, Washington, D.C. 1964.

Breast

BARASH, I.M., et al.: Quantitative thermography as a predictor of breast cancer. Cancer (Philad.) **31**, (4), 769–776 (1973).

BLOOM, H.: The influence of delay in the natural history and prognosis of breast cancer. Brit. J. Cancer **19**, 228–262 (1965).

CLEMMESEN, J.: Statistical studies in malignant neoplasms. II Tables. Acta path. microbiol. scand., Suppl. **174** (1965).

EGAN, R.L.: Mammography. American Lecture Series, Publ. No. 568.

EGAN, R.L.: Present status of mammography. Ann. N.Y. Acad. Sci. **114**, 794–802 (1964).

GERSHON-COHEN, J., BOREADIS-BORDEN, A.G.: Detection of unsuspected breast cancer by mammography. Ann. N.Y. Acad. Sci. **114**, 782–793 (1964).

Seventh Annual Seminar: The detection of early cancer of the breast. Cancer (Philad.) **23** (4), (1969).

SHAPIRO, S., STRAX, P., VENET, L.: Evaluation of the role of periodic breast screening in reducing the mortality from breast cancer, J. Amer. med. Ass. **215**, 1777–1785 (1971).

SHIMKIN, M.: The numerical method in therapeutic medicine. Publ. Hlth Rep. (Wash.) **79**, 1–12 (1963).

STRAX, P. et al.: Mammography and clinical examination in mass screening for cancer of the breast. Cancer (Philad.) **20**, 2184–2188 (1967).

VENET, L., et al.: Adequacies and inadequacies of breast examinations by physicians in mass screening. Cancer (Philad.) 28, 1546–1551 (1971).

WOLFE, J.N.: Mammography as a screening examination in breast cancer. Radiology 84, 703–708 (1965).

Female Genital

AHLUWALIA, H., DOLL, R.: Mortality from cancer of the cervix uteri in British Columbia and other parts of Canada. Brit. J. prev. soc. Med. 22, 161–164 (1968).

ANTOINE, T.: Amer. J. Obstet. Gynec. 68, 466 (1964).

BOYES, D., et al.: Results of treatment of 4389 cases of preclinical cervical squamous carcinoma. J. Obstet. Gynec. Cwlth 77, 769–772 (1970).

BOYES, D.A., FIDLER, H.K.: Symposium on Cancer of the Uterus, U.I.C.C. Rev. Inst. Nacional de Cancer, Mexico, Sept. 1964, p. 456.

CHRISTOPHERSON, W., et al.: Cervix cancer control in Louisville, Kentucky. Cancer (Philad.) 26, 29–38 (1970).

FIDLER, H., et al.: Cervical cytology in the control of cancer of the cervic. Mod. Med. 25, 9–15 (1970).

JOHNSON, Lurna: The histopathological approach to early cervical neoplasia. Obstet. gynec. Surv. 24, 735–767 (1969).

KAISER, R.F., INGRAHAM, S.C., HILBERG, A.W.: Publ. Hlth Rep. (Wash.) 75, 523 (1960).

PAPANICOLAOU, G.N., TRAUT, H.: Diagnosis of uterine cancer by the vaginal smear. New York: Commonwealth Found 1943.

Stockholm Committee: 15th Annual Report 1973

Male Genital

BOYER, W.F.: Carcinoma of the prostate. A cytological study. J. Urol. (Baltimore) 63, 234–345 (1950).

CLEMMESEN, J.: The testis. Statistical studies in malignant neoplasms. III. Acta path. microbiol. scand. (1968).

CREEVEY, C.D.: The diagnosis and treatment of early carcinoma of the prostate. J. Amer. med. Ass. 120, 1102–1105 (1948).

DARGET, R.: Le cancer de la prostate. Paris: Masson & Cie. 1958.

DIXON, F.J., MOORE, R.A.: Tumors of the male sex organs. Armed Forces, Ins. of Pathology, Sect. VIII, fasc. 31 b–32, 127–142 (1952).

DVOŘÁK, V., GROSS, K., STARA, B.: Aspiration punction cytology on oncological practice. Acta Un. int. Cancr. 3, 807–810 (1964).

FERGUSON, R.S.: Diagnosis and treatment of early carcinoma of the prostate. J. Urol. (Baltimore) 37, 774–782 (1937).

GROSS, K., ČAPEK, J., ŠVÁB, L.: Cytodiagnostic of the prostate and urinary bladder's tumours. Prakt. Lék. (Praha) 42, 15–16 (1962).

HERBUT, P.A., LUBIN, E.N.: Cancer cells in prostatic secretions. J. Urol. (Baltimore) 57, 542–551 (1947).

NIEBURGS, H.E.: Cytologic technics. New York and London: Grune & Stratton 1956.

O'DONNELL, W.E., DAY, E., VENET, L.: Early detection and diagnosis of cancer. St. Louis: C.V. Mosby Co. 1962.

PETERS, H.: The prostatic smear. Cancer (Philad.) 3, 481–487 (1950).

Bladder

BALOGH, F., SZENDRÓI, Z.: Pathologie und Klinik der Nierengeschwülste. Budapest: Verlag der ungarischen Akademie 1960.

CAMPBELL, M.: Urology, vol. II. Philadelphia and London: W.B. Saunders Co. 1954.

FRANKSSON, C.: Tumors of the urinary bladder. A pathological and clinical study of 434 cases. Acta chir. scand., Suppl. 151 (1950).

GROSS, K., ČAPEK, J., ŠVÁD, L.: Cytodiagnostic of the prostate and urinary bladder's tumours. Prakt. Lék. (Praha) 42, 15–16 (1962).

JAMES, A.G.: Cancer prognosis manual. American Cancer Society Inc., 1967.

JEWETT, H.: Tumours of the bladder, Urology, 3rd ed. vol. 2. Philadelphia: W.B. Saunders & Co., 1970.

KAVECKA, M.: Cytodiagnostika Raka. Warszawa: Panstwony Zakad, Wydawnictw Lekarskich 1956.

NIEBURGS, H.E.: Cytologic technics. New York and London: Grune & Stratton 1956.

O'DONNELL, W.E., DAY, E., VENET, L.: Early detection and diagnosis of cancer. St. Louis: C.V. Mosby Co. 1962.

PAPANICOLAOU, G.N.: Cytology of the urine sediment in neoplasms of the urinary tract. J. Urol. (Baltimore) 57, 375–379 (1947).

TROLL, W.: Studies on the nature of proximal bladder carcinogens. Bladder Cancer-a Symposium. Birmingham, Alabama: Aesculapius Publ. Co., 1967.

Skin

HABER, H.: Cytodiagnosis in dermatology. Brit. J. Derm. 66, 79–94 (1954).

HITCH, J.M., et al.: Evaluation of rapid method of cytologic diagnosis in suspected skin cancer. Sth. med. J. (Bgham, Ala.) 44, 407–414 (1951).

KLEIN, E., et al.: Tumours of the skin. J. Surg. Oncol. 3, 331–337 (1971).

LEVER, W.: Histopathology of the skin. Philadelphia: J.B. Lippincott 1967.

TRAENKLE, H.L., BURKE, E.M.: Curettement technic for biopsy. Use in detection of cutaneous cancer. J. Amer. med. Ass. 143, 429 (1950).

URBACH, F., et al.: Ultraviolet radiation and skin cancer in man. Advances in biology of skin, vol. VII. Oxford: Pergamon Press 1966.

WILSON, G.T.: Cutaneous smears. A diagnostic aid in certain malignant lesions of the skin. J. invest. Derm. **22**, 173–187 (1954).

Thyroid

ANGEVINE, D.M., JABLON, S.: Late irradiation of neoplasia and other disease in Japan. Ann. N.Y. Acad. Sci. **114**, 823–831 (1964).

BOEHME, E.J., WINSHIP, T., LINDSAY, S., KYPRIADIS, G.: An evaluation of needle biopsy of the thyroid gland. Surg. Gynec. Obstet. **119**, 831–834 (1964).

CLARK, D.E.: Association of irradiation with cancer of the thyroid in children and adolescents. J. Amer. med. Ass. **159**, 1007–1009 (1955).

EDDINGER, C.: Histological classification of tumours of the thyroid gland. Geneva, W.H.O. in print.

LINDSAY, S.: Carcinoma of the thyroid gland. Springfield (Ill.): Ch. C. Thomas 1960.

SEGI, M., KURIHARA, M.: Cancer mortality for selected sites in 24 countries, No. 3, 1960/61. Dept. of Public Health, Sendai, Japan 1964.

WARREN, S., MEISSNER, W.A.: tumours of the thyroid gland. Atlas of tumor pathology, A.F.I.P. 1963.

All Sites

Cancer. Vols. 1–6 (RAVEN, R.W.). London: Butterworth & Co. Ltd. 1957.

Cancer incidence in five continents. UICC Report. Berlin, New York: Springer 1970.

Cancer medicine. Philadelphia: Lea & Febinger 1973.

Cancer mortality in 24 countries (SEGI, M. and KURIHARA, M.). Nagoya: Japan Cancer Society 1972.

End results in cancer—No. 4. U.S. Dept. of Health, Education & Welfare. Bethesda: National Institute of Health, 1973.

Screening in medical care. Nuffield Hospitals Trust. London: Oxford University Press 1968.

Chapter III

Planning Cancer Detection Programmes

It is obvious from the previous chapter that there may be difficulties in implementing cancer detection techniques as control measures applied to populations at large; doubts may also arise as to the likely benefit from such procedures. This chapter presents the main questions to be answered before a cancer detection programme is instituted; these questions can conveniently be considered under the headings:

1. Importance of the disease to be controlled.

2. Knowledge of its natural history.

3. Effectiveness of the detection procedure.

4. Effectiveness of the treatment resources.

5. Operational problems in setting up a screening programme.

1. Importance of the Disease to be Controlled

Since a cancer detection programme involves examining apparently healthy people of which only a small proportion would be shown to harbour a cancerous or precancerous lesion, it is difficult to justify examination, except of those sites which constitute a major problem. In general, the severity of a cancer problem in a population is determined by mortality and incidence levels; but other considerations, such as response to treatment, may influence the decision.

Each country has to establish its own priorities because of the variable geographical distribution of cancer. Table I, based on data for 24 selected countries compiled by SEGI, shows the range between highest and lowest standardized mortality rates for selected sites. On this basis, for instance, stomach cancer is clearly significant in Japan, with higher rates for both sexes, but of much

Table I. Range in standardized mortality rates for selected sites of cancer (SEGI, 1966–1967)

Site	Highest rate	Country	Lowest rate	Country
Male				
Buccal cavity	10.0	France	1.3	Japan
Stomach	66.8	Japan	8.5	U.S.A. (whites)
Intestine	15.4	Scotland	3.5	Japan
Larynx	10.7	France	0.5	Sweden
Lung	78.1	Scotland	10.9	Portugal
Prostate	29.5	Sweden	1.5	Japan
Female				
Buccal cavity	2.0	N. Ireland	0.5	Germany (F.R.)
Stomach	34.6	Japan	4.4	U.S.A. (whites)
Intestine	15.0	Scotland	3.4	Japan
Lung	11.7	Scotland	2.7	Portugal
Breast	26.5	Netherlands	4.0	Japan
Uterus	22.2	U.S.A. (non-whites)	5.0	Israel

Table II. Range in standardized incidence rates for selected sites of cancer. Five continents, UICC, 1970

Site	Highest rate	Country	Lowest rate	Country
		Male		
Buccal cavity	7.8	Puerto Rico	0.5	Germany (DDR)
Stomach	95.0	Japan	8.0	Nigeria
Colon	19.3	Canada	3.6	Colombia
Lung	70.0	Finland	13.6	Puerto Rico
Prostate	40.1	New Zealand	3.7	Japan
		Female		
Stomach	24.8	Colombia	9.5	New Zealand (white)
Colon	20.8	U.S.A. (whites)	0.9	Nigeria
Breast	56.1	U.S.A. (whites)	13.7	Nigeria
Cervix	76.0	Colombia	4.9	Israel (Jews)
Uterus	15.0	Canada	1.5	India

less consequence for the U.S. white population; breast cancer in women presents a far larger problem in the Netherlands than in Japan.

Where incidence data are available these can be used to establish priorities. Table II shows the range in the incidence rates (taken from Cancer in Five Continents).

In both Tables I and II the contrasts are shown by standardized rates which, taking into account differences in population structure, provide a measure of the relative risks in the different countries. Such measures may not be the most informative. A country may have a higher standardized rate for a particular site, but because the population is relatively young the cancer will not be one of the most common causes of death. On the other hand, a country like Scotland has a high proportion of old people and the highest standardized death rate for lung cancer, so that its problem is even greater than is indicated by the figure in Table I. For many developing countries it might be more appropriate to use proportional mortality, i.e. the proportion

$$\frac{\text{Death from specific Ca}}{\text{Death from all causes}}$$

as a measure of priority rather than standardized rates.

2. Knowledge of Natural History

Detection will sometimes be aimed at so-called precancerous lesions, e.g. leukoplakia for oral cancer, carcinoma *in situ* for cervical cancer, or at early invasive cancer, e.g. in the breast. The potential value of detection in cancer control depends on the relationship between these lesions and progressive invasive cancer. The value of detecting leukoplakia would clearly be greater if it always preceded oral cancer than if it occurred as an antecedent in only a small proportion. Some of the debate on the effectiveness of cervical cytology initiates such an argument. It is postulated that carcinoma *in situ* usually develops several years before there is progression to invasive cancer, and hence there is reasonable opportunity to detect the early stage by cytological examination. If, however, the carcinoma *in situ* stage is short, the lesion would often be missed and the screening procedure could operate only at the level of discovering invasive cancer. Furthermore, if a proportion of the cases of carcinoma *in situ* did not progress further or regressed to normal, a number of patients in whom this was detected would be submitted to treatment unnecessarily.

It is difficult to produce the evidence which would dispose of these doubts satisfactorily. A direct measure of the progression from normal → dysplasia → carcinoma *in situ* → invasive cancer could only be obtained by repeated examination of the same individuals at frequent intervals to be reasonably certain of detecting a short carcinoma *in situ* stage. Even then, the finding of carcinoma *in situ* would lead to the excision of the lesion, and nothing could be learned of its progression or regression if untreated. Follow-up studies of this kind are being carried out. In Cheshire a computer-based screening programme provides for re-examination of women at various intervals after their original test in order to provide estimates of incidence of the cytological positive state. The relationship between this positive state and invasive cancer will probably have to be obtained indirectly by inference from other data, and studies of this kind are also in progress (KNOX, 1973).

For the present, screening programmes will at times have to operate in ignorance of the natural history of the condition to be controlled. It would be advantageous, therefore, to design programmes so that they can yield such information, which could be used to improve future performance.

3. Effectiveness of the Detection Procedure

A detection procedure suitable for population use should be relatively simple and inexpensive. The aim is usually to discover persons warranting further investigation by more refined diagnostic methods rather than to establish the final diagnosis. It is particularly important that the screening test be *sensitive*, picking up as much as possible all those with abnormalities. In other words, the test should not give false negative results, i.e. an apparently clean bill of health to a person with abnormality.

It is further desirable that the screening test be *specific*, primarily picking up only those with the specified abnormality. It should not give false positive results, i.e. an indication of abnormality in someone not suffering from the disease in question. To some extent, failure of specificity is more acceptable than poor sensitivity; but the degree of anxiety caused to the person with a false positive result, and the risk of unnecessary investigation and treatment must be borne in mind. False positives may add to the load placed on diagnostic service, another factor which may determine whether a test is sufficiently specific.

Some tests might appear to have acceptable degrees of sensitivity and specificity in the hands of some workers, but behave less satisfactorily elsewhere. Differences may be systematic, one person's results being consistently higher or lower than another's, or irregular, so that the reproducibility of the test varies. In either situation the value of the test will be diminished; the aim should be to achieve consistency in each operator or laboratory over a period of time, as well as consistency among the various operators and laboratories.

The issue of reproducibility will have to be resolved separately for each detection programme, whereas the question of sensitivity and specificity applies more generally and can often be settled by reference to previous studies. The following examples illustrate how this may be done.

Increasing attention is being paid to the error rate in cervical cytology, since it is recognised that error can occur both in the collection of the specimen and in its analysis. In the Cheshire screening programme, referred to earlier, two examinations are made on each woman within the relatively short interval of three months to enable measuring the frequency of discrepancies. From previous experience it is estimated that this may be about 20%.

A measure of reproducibility was sought in the Montreal studies using the Farr test for carcino-embryonic antigen (CEA). A number of duplicate samples were tested in local laboratories and in the Montreal laboratory, yielding the following results:

Table III. Comparison of CEA levels from duplicate samples examined in the Montreal laboratory and the local laboratories. (Canad. med. Ass. J./July 8, 1972/Vol. 107)

CEA levels (ng/ml) in local laboratories	CEA levels (ng/ml) in Montreal laboratory					
	< 1.0	1.0–2.4	2.5–4.9	5.0–9.9	10.0–19.9	20.0 or more
< 1.0	136	52	32	5	—	3
1.0–2.4	36	8	13	3	1	—
2.5–4.9	24	32	29	8	1	—
5.0–9.9	9	5	13	12	5	—
10.0–19.9	7	1	3	9	13	11
20.0 or more	10	4	8	5	10	23

It can be seen that 221 of the 531 pairs (within the diagonals) yielded identical results, and a further 189 differed by only one class (e.g. 36 samples were estimated in Montreal to have less than 1.0 ng/ml but 1.0–2.4 ng/ml in local laboratories). If a 'positive' result was arbitrarily defined as 2.5 ng/ml or more, the table could be re-cast as follows:

Local laboratories	Montreal laboratory		
	Negative < 2.5 ng/ml	Positive 2.5+ng/ml	
Negative < 2.5 ng/ml	232	57	289 (54.4%)
Positive 2.5+ng/ml	150	242	242 (45.6%)
Total	324 (61%)	207 (39.0%)	531 (100%)

It is clear that in this instance, although the overall proportion of positives was not greatly different, 39% by the Montreal and 46% by the local laboratories, 149 of the 531 samples, over a quarter, were differently classified. A greater degree of reproducibility would usually be demanded for a population-based detection programme.

A different order of reproducibility was seen in a study of the alpha foetoprotein test in the detection of primary liver cancer. In this investigation, three laboratories tested

813 sera independently and blindly and were in complete agreement for 786 (94.7%). This is a high degree of reproducibility, a level which may not be easy to achieve with other detection procedures.

Sensitivity and specificity can also be estimated from the CEA and alpha foetoprotein studies. Taking the same definition of a positive result for CEA of 2.5 or more ng/ml, the following results were obtained in the Montreal laboratory in:

Test result	Colo-rectal cancer	"Other" diagnoses	All patients
Negative < 2.5 ng/ml	44 (38.2%)	209 (67.1%)	253
Positive 2.5+ng/ml	71 (61.8%)	102 (32.9%)	173
Total	115	311	426

It can be seen that at the 2.5 ng/ml level only 62% of colo-rectal cancer gave a positive result, which was also given by as much as 33% of those with other diagnosis; the test at this level was neither particularly sensitive nor specific.

Proportions of this kind are often used as quantitative measurement of these characteristics, and can be expressed in general terms as:

Sensitivity % =

$$\frac{\text{No. with positive test result}}{\text{No. with disease under investigation}} \times 100$$

Specificity % =

$$\frac{\text{No. with negative test result}}{\text{No. without disease under investigation}} \times 100$$

Turning again to the alpha foetoprotein study, a positive result was obtained in 151 of 231 cases of liver cancer, a sensitivity of 65.4%. A negative result was obtained in 541 of the 555 controls with other dieseases, a very high degree of specificity, 97.8%.

Table IV. Effectiveness of treatment for selected sites of cancer. (End Results in Cancer, No. 4, U.S. Dept. of Health, Education and Welfare)

Site	Male (%)		Female (%)	
	5 yr	10 yr	5 yr	10 yr
Lip	87	82	89	81
Mouth	40	30	54	38
Stomach	10	10	14	11
Colon	43	38	47	42
Lung	8	5	12	9
Breast	—	—	63	48
Cervix	—	—	59	54
Corpus	—	—	72	68
Prostate	52	32	—	—
Bladder	57	50	56	49

4. Effectiveness of Treatment

The establishment of a detection programme presupposes that the patients discovered to have abnormalities can be fully investigated and treated, and that they will benefit from treatment. Each centre has to consider the sufficiency of its own diagnostic and treatment facilities in the light of the expected yield of new cases. The question of the advantages of early treatment to the patient, however, can often be decided generally from experience elsewhere. One of the prime measures of success of treatment is survival. Data on 5-year survival rates by site are available from a number of sources. Although these are based on different populations, these rates are fairly uniform and any one set of data can be used as a general guide to the probabilities of survival. Table IV below shows selected data from End Results in Cancer, Report No. 4, which are based on the experience of more than 100 hospitals in different parts of the United States.

From this information it is clear that detection of cancer of the bronchus could not be expected to lead to markedly improved survival; because even if it were possible to ascertain cases with localized disease only, the 5-year survival rate would be less than 30% for those patients, and worse for those with more extensive disease. For many other sites the expectation would be far more optimistic, particularly since a detection programme should pick up a high proportion of early cases.

Although the value of detection and treatment is usually considered largely in terms of survival, there are other benefits from early ascertainment which might be wise to take into account. The management of a patient who presents himself for the first time with advanced disease can present formidable problems, e.g. with fistulae that may not be possible to resolve satisfactorily. The same patient seen earlier might have been protected from some of the more distressing complications, even though the question of ultimate survival was not altered. The impact on the patient's quality of life may be a significant consideration for a detection programme.

5. Operational Problems of Setting up a Screening Programme

By nature, a detection programme has to provide for the examination of a large number of persons, the majority of whom will not be suffering from cancer. The case for setting up a programme is well-grounded because: cancer is an important community problem, there is a good case for early detection, and a suitable test is available. The critical question may then be the size and nature of the resources needed to mount the programme. The problem of providing reliable testing facilities has been considered in a previous section; the priority for using such resources for detection is a separate issue. For example, the HIP study of screening for breast cancer by mammography and clinical examination, which is refered to later in more detail, has made a case for such examination; but its implementation elsewhere may be limited because large-scale mammography would be too demanding on existing diagnostic radiographic services.

A reduction in the resources needed for detection can sometimes be achieved by restricting the activity to sections of the population most in need. For example, because the yield of positive results would be small and the risk of cervical cancer is minimal,

cytology would not be of much value to a population of younger women or to programmes that customarily set a lower limit for eligibility, e.g. 30 years of age. The same principle can be extended, as far as it is possible, to define risk groups. For cervical cancer a relationship between mortality and socio-economic factors has been demonstrated, which may in part be a reflection of the women's sexual activity. A similar correlation has recently been shown between the prevalence of carcinoma *in situ* and the husband's occupation.

This information suggests that certain socio-economic groups should have priority in screening programmes; furthermore, the similarity in epidemiological behaviour adds to the evidence that carcinoma in situ is an important stage in the development of invasive cancer and is worth detecting.

Table V. Relationship of carcinoma in situ and occupation of husband. (J. WAKEFIELD *et al.*: Brit. med. J. **1973 II**, 142)

Occupational orders	No. of Women	No. positive per 1,000	S.M.R.*
Professional, technical workers and artists (XXV)	37,700	4.11	42
Leather workers (IX)	811	4.93	103†
Clerical workers (XXI)	28,013	6.00	67
Electrical and electronic workers (VI)	11,588	7.08	92
Makers of other products—rubber, plastics etc. (XIV)	2,770	7.58	88
Administrators and managers (XXIV)	14,659	8.12	50
Farmers, foresters, fishermen (I)	4,645	8.40	93
Paper and printing workers (XIII)	4,067	8.61	66†
Food, drink, and tobacco workers (XII)	3,571	8.96	117
Clothing workers (XI)	2,178	9.18	79†
Woodworkers (VIII)	6,466	9.28	77
Gas, coke, and chemical workers (III)	4,861	9.87	123
Engineering and allied trades workers not elsewhere classified (VII)	47,108	10.02	96
Sales workers (XXII)	21,796	10.41	71
Glass and ceramics makers (IV)	863	11.59	84†
Textile workers (X)	3,121	11.86	146
Armed Forces, British and Foreign (XXVI)	1,588	11.96	102
Service, sport, and recreation workers (XXIII)	14,542	12.17	112
Warehousemen, storekeepers, packers, and bottlers (XX)	5,018	12.36	81
Transport and communications workers (XIX)	26,631	13.18	145
Drivers of stationary engines, cranes, etc. (XVII)	3,045	13.46	150
Furnace, forge, foundry, rolling mill workers (V)	1,738	13.81	111
Painters and decorators (XVI)	4,175	14.37	111
Construction workers (XV)	8,436	14.94	118
Miners and quarrymen (II)	2,170	15.67	133
Labourers not elsewhere classified (XVIII)	12,351	17.73	186

Providing there is sufficient knowledge of the epidemiology of a cancer, it may be possible to define risk groups on which it would be worth concentrating the activities of a detection programme. The nature of these risk factors may be varied. Some that indicate persons at low risk who do not require attention may be just as useful as others that point to high risk. For example, if a detection programme was appropriate for cancer of the lung, non-smokers could be excluded. Results may be related to personal habits like smoking, or to others, such as: chewing of betel, associated with oral cancer; occupational exposure, as in the bladder cancer of workers with Benzpyrene; some environmental exposure, as in the skin cancer of fair-skinned inhabitants of sunny countries, bladder cancer where schistomiasis is common; or in the special liability exemplified by the relatively frequent occurrence of large gut cancer in patients with previous polyposis or ulcerative colitis.

However, experience in cervical cytology shows that epidemiological definition of a risk group is not enough because the less-educated and lower socio–economic groups with the higher risk usually come forward for examination less readily than those at lesser risk. One of the major tasks of a detection activity may be to ensure that it reaches those most in need, and in this the role of education may be critical.

An alternative approach to reducing the size of the population to be screened in breast cancer is offered by the detection of abnormal urinary steroid patterns in patients suffering from the disease (BULBROOK et al.). This finding is being extended by surveying a general population to determine its possible use as a risk group on which other techniques, such as mammography, could be concentrated.

The timing and frequency of examination are important in a detection programme, influencing both its likelihood for success and its practical application. Detection does not firmly categorize a patient's status; tests have to be repeated at suitable intervals as long as the person remains at risk. The choice of interval should be related to knowledge of the incidence rate of new lesions; in deciding on an interval, we must compromise between, on the one hand, re-examinationing often enough to ensure that a new lesion arising since the previous test has not advanced too far, and on the other hand, not overburdening the patient or the medical facilities. Little attention has been paid to this problem beyond determining age limits, as was done for cervical cytology; and further investigation is required. For the present, little guidance can be given; we can simply emphasize that whatever decisions are made, the programme should have an efficient system of recalling patients for re-examination, and good record system to ensure that all information on an individual patient, whenever he is seen, is kept together.

In the preceding sections, a number of factors have been mentioned that will affect the success of detection in cancer control and the demand on resources made by the programme: the natural history of the disease; the suitability of the test procedure in regard to sensitivity, specificity, and reproducibility, and requirements for staff and equipment; the frequency of re-examination desired; the treatment facilities available and their estimated effectiveness; the possibility of recognising high-risk groups and concentrating activity on them; and the response of the population to the programme. Each of these could in turn provide a choice of alternative plans, e.g. between re-examination at 1-, 5-, or 10-year intervals, between attempts to cover a whole population or to concentration on some part of it; each of these choices could be the subject of separate investigation. The combined effect of these alternative procedures would, however, form a complex pattern that could not be resolved by a simple experiment. In this situation, guidance may be sought by formulating a mathematical model of the activity that relates its separate parts. It should also simulate the outcome (predict results) given different data on such elements as: incidence of abnormality, test error, interval between examinations, etc.) A model of this kind related to cervical cytology and some predictions which arise from the simulation are described by KNOX (1973).

Evaluation of Cancer Detection

Every public health activity, such as cancer control, requires evaluation to ensure that it is operating as required and is achieving the intended results. Without such appraisal much time and effort can be wasted. The end results, in terms of increased survival or in improved quality of life, as a rule can be measured only by reference to large populations and may require elaborate ad hoc studies. This type of evaluation cannot be built into every programme. On the other hand, no detection programme should operate without measuring:

The reproducibility and accuracy of its testing procedure;

The yield obtained from different sections of the population;

The extent to which different sections are covered, an estimate of the number and type of non-responders;

The relapse rate for re-examination;

The outcome, in terms of cancer incidence and mortality, among the screened population, an estimate of these for the non-responders.

On the more general issue of the effectiveness of detection as a control measure there is substantial evidence available on some procedures and very little for others. There are several kinds of such evidence, regarding: the proportion of early cases discovered, the trends in mortality and morbidity since detection activities started, and comparisons between screened and unscreened populations. Most of the results come from observations of the situation as it developed since detection; only a small part cames from specially designed evaluation studies.

The experience of British Columbia with screening for cancer of the cervix is partic-

ularly valuable because the programme started as long ago as 1949 and now covers 80% of the female population over 20 years of age. In this project there is one central laboratory providing uniform reporting of cytology. The mortality and incidence data are collated with the help of the Division of Vital Statistics of the Province of British Columbia and a registry for these two rates is maintained in the laboratory.

The trend of mortality for squamous carcinoma of the cervix and incidence of clinical invasive carcinoma in women over 20 years of age in British Columbia for the fourteen years between 1958–1971 is shown in Table VI.

These rates indicate a general decline in mortality, particularly when the earlier period 1958–1964 is compared with the later period 1965–1971. The decline in incidence has been far more striking, with recent rates only about a half those at the beginning of the period.

Doubts have been raised concerning the interpretation of the mortality trend in British Columbia because other Canadian Provinces and western countries in which screening by cervical cytology has been used much less also have falling rates. Aluwalia and Doll have compared the trends in a

Table VI. British Columbia, squamous carcinoma of the cervix rates per 100,000 women over 20 years of age

Year	Mortality	Incidence
1958	11.4	23.7
1959	10.6	22.6
1960	9.9	19.7
1961	10.25	23.2
1962	12.9	15.5
1963	11.0	19.1
1964	10.6	16.3
1965	7.7	14.7
1966	7.8	13.6
1967	6.4	14.3
1968	8.8	13.0
1969	7.1	13.9
1970	6.9	12.3
1971	8.1	10.7

Table VII. Comparison of screened and unscreened population in British Columbia-Squamous carcinoma of cervix

| Year | Population | | Rates per 100,000 women over 20 years of age | | | |
| | Screened (%) | Unscreened (%) | Mortality | | Incidence | |
			Screened	Unscreened	Screened	Unscreened
1962	32.5	67.5	1.2	18.6	4.3	21.0
1963	42.0	58.0	0.9	18.4	4.7	29.5
1964	49.5	50.5	1.5	19.5	4.6	27.8
1965	56.0	44.0	0.6	17.2	4.2	28.8
1966	63.0	37.0	1.3	18.6	4.8	28.6
1967	68.0	32.0	1.2	17.6	5.4	33.4
1968	73.0	27.0	1.7	27.8	4.4	36.5
1969	78.0	22.0	1.8	25.8	3.4	51.4

number of countries and have concluded that the British Columbia rates probably are simply beginning to show a favourable response that may be related to the screening programme.

Table VII compares the experience of the screened and unscreened population of women over 20 years old in British Columbia, in terms of mortality and incidence of clinical invasive carcinoma.

Over this period 1962–1969 shown in the Table the proportion of the female population which was screened rose from just over 30% to nearly 80%; the incidence in this period has not altered much in either direction; mortality, though it shows a possible increase, has remained very low. By contrast, the incidence and mortality have increased in the unscreened population, particularly in the last few years; and both rates are considerably higher than those in the screened women—mortality by a factor of more than 10, incidence by about sixfold.

These contrasts cannot be taken at face value as direct estimates of the impact of screening because the screened population is inevitably selected in some way. The factors included in such selection are difficult to determine; but it might reasonably be assumed that among the women who did not participate there may be a number at high risk. This could explain the rising mortality and incidence among the unscreened

group, which as it gets smaller contains a larger proportion of hardcore non-responders.

Selection could account for some of the contrast between screened and unscreened sections; however, that the same or even greater differences between the rates has been maintained over a period in which the relative size of the two populations has altered so profoundly, suggests that there is a real difference in risk. This view is reinforced by the comparison shown in Table VIII, demonstrating that in the period 1961–1970 the proportion of Stage-1 cases among the clinical invasive cancers is much higher in the screened than the unscreened cases.

A somewhat similar picture emerges from another large cervical cytology programme in Louisville, Kentucky. The programme began in Jefferson County in the city of

Table VIII. Proportions of invasive cases by stage for screened and unscreened populations

Stage	Screened (%)	Unscreened (%)
I	38.7	24.7
II	35.3	35.4
III	21.3	28.2
IV	2.7	7.5
Not known	2.0	4.2
Total	100.0	100.0

Louisville in 1956, and by 1967 over 90% of the adult female population had been screened at least once. The rate of discovery of newly diagnosed carcinoma *in situ* increased from 9.4 per 100,000 women 20 years and over in 1953–1955 to 59.2 per 100,000 in 1965–1967. Over this period the incidence of invasive squamous carcinoma rose at first, possibly because of better ascertainment, but later declined, so that the 1965–1967 rates were about 30% lower than those in 1953–1955. At the same time the proportion of Stage-I cases about doubled, from 32% to 57% of cases. These trends were found in both Caucasians and Non-Caucasians and in most age groups—except for the older women in whom screening had reached a smaller porportion. A comparison of mortality showed that there had been a decrease in Jefferson County from 1953 to 1967, in contrast to very little change in the state of Kentucky as a whole, where there had been no mass screening.

Suggestions on a favourable trend that could be related to large-scale screening for stomach cancer came from Japan, where this cancer is particularly significant.

Mass screening began in 1953 and has developed to the point that over 2 million adults, mostly over the age of 40, are examined annually by radiological techniques. In Kanagawri Prefecture in the years 1962–1968, the mortality rates per 100,0000 were 97.6 for screened and 121.1 for unscreened persons. In the country as a whole, mortality declined, particularly in the Prefectures where extensive screening had been carried out; it was also observed that the 5-year survival rate was over 90% for early cases.

Observations like those described above, in connection with cervical and stomach cancer, give some indication of the probable success of detection. However, they can never be entirely free of the criticism that such trends also would have occurred without screening, or that screened populations were self-selected and by nature less at risk of developing cancer. The method of evaluation exempt from such criticism is the randomized control trial. A good example of this method is provided in a study set up by the Health Insurance Plan (HIP) in New York to evaluate mammography and provide clinical examination to detect breast cancer.

In this study, set up in 1963, women aged 40 to 64 years were randomly allocated to two groups, the *study* group to be screened annually and the *control* group to use the ordinary medical care services; there were 31,000 women in each sample. The two samples were shown to be comparable in respect to age, religion, education, marital status, number of pregnancies, and factors which might have been relevant to the risk of breast

Table IX. Breast cancer detection rates, 5 years of observation from date of entry

Population	Breast cancers	
	No.	Rate per 1,000[a]
Study-screened		
Detection due to initial examined [b]	55	2.72
Detection due to annual reexamination	77	1.51
Detection not due to screening [c]	91	0.92
Study-refused screening	73	1.37
Control	284	1.86
Study	296	

[a] 20,211 women had initial screening examination.

[b] Includes only cases diagnosed in course of regular medical care; case detection not due to follow-up of screening findings.

[c] Rate of detection due to initial screening is per 1,000 women examined; other rates are per 1,000 person-years.

Table X. Breast cancer deaths by interval from start of observation to end of 5 years of follow-up

Interval since start of observation[a]	No. of person-years		No. of breast cancer deaths	
	Control	Study	Control	Study[b]
Total	152,742	151,660	63	40
First two years	61,781	61,337	8	11
Third year	30,567	30,350	12	6
Fourth year	30,327	30,114	18	8
Fifth year	30,067	29,859	25	15

[a] Starting point is date of entry to study or control group.
[b] Includes women screened and women who refused screening.

cancer. After 5 years of follow-up, 296 breast cancers were diagnosed in the study group and 284 in the control group. The method of detection and the corresponding rates are shown in Table IX.

The relatively low rate of breast cancer in the group not accepting screening examinations suggests that study women with a high risk for such cancer tended to self-select themselves for screening. Clinical and mammography examinations contributed independently to the detection of breast cancer, about 30% by mammography alone, 40% by clinical examination alone, and 30% by both techniques. Mammography contributed much less in younger women, 40–49 years of age, than in those over 50. A high proportion, 70% of the cancers detected by screening, had no histological evidence of axillary node involvement, compared with 52% for cancers in the screened study group not detected due to screening, 40% for cancers in those who refused screening, and 46% for cancers in the control group.

In terms of mortality, the control and study groups were similar for the first two years of observation; but in each of the next three years, deaths in the study group were about half those in the control. When examined separately by age, the screened population appeared to be like the study group at 40–49 years, but showed lower rates for the older women.

The 5-year fatality rate in confirmed breast cancer cases also indicates an advan-

tage in the study group, where it was 28%, compared to 42% in the controls. In the study group, the fatality rate in cases occurring in the screened women was lower than that in women who refused screening; this difference is consistent with the observation on the proportions with lymph node involvement.

Studies of this kind are very demanding and not easily repeated. Their particular value is in the unequivocal way they can answer precise questions on the effect of a screening programme. The HIP study is particularly significant in providing clear evidence that a well-designed screening programme has saved lives.

Table XI. Breast cancer deaths by age at death, 5 years of follow-up

Age at death	Breast cancer deaths			
	Number		Rate per 10,000 person-years	
	Control	Study[a]	Control	Study[a]
Total	63	40	4.1	2.6
40–49 years	12	13	2.4	2.5
(40–44)	(2)	(1)	—	—
(45–49)	(10)	(12)	—	—
50–59 years	34	16	5.0	2.3
(50–54)	(16)	(9)	—	—
(55–59)	(18)	(7)	—	—
60–69 years	17	11	5.0	3.4

[a] Includes women screened and women who refused screening.

Chapter IV

Social and Educational Factors in Cancer Detection

The major communicable diseases can, to a large extent, be controlled by legislation and vigorous public health measures; and for at least one major, killing form of cancer, prevention is perfectly feasible if people can be persuaded or obliged to give up heavy cigarette smoking. However, it can be said with some truth of most forms of cancer, that until the introduction of effective screening tests, the patient was responsible for the first vital step in diagnosis—deciding that some symptom called for a visit to his doctor. To a large extent this is still true. Tests that are both economically and clinically practicable are not yet available for the early detection of all forms of cancer; and the tests that are practicable are either not yet available in all countries, or have not yet become regarded as an acceptable routine by the population at risk.

Public education must therefore be an integral part of programmes of cancer detection and must have two objectives: (1) to persuade people to seek prompt medical advice when certain warning signs appear; and (2) to encourage them, particularly those at high risk, to take part in screening programmes. The first involves influencing the usual habits of seeking medical care in a given community, as well as changing prevailing attitudes toward cancer. The second calls for a single precisely defined course of action (attendance for examination) as a means of preventing cancer from developing or, at least, of progressing beyond the reach of curative treatment.

Neither of these two educational problems can be tackled in isolation. They demand a proper appreciation of the difficulties involved in trying to counter the powerful social pressures that influence people to conform to well-established patterns of behaviour. These problems require an awareness of the need to move by small steps, expecting no sudden major change in the established habits or beliefs of the community. Perhaps one of the most attractive changes we can offer, from the point of view of the man in the street, is for him to be able to accept some forms of cancer as preventable, in the sense that they can now be found and dealt with as precancerous lesions. Motives causing people to go to physicians have been studied far too little; it has been suggested that some go for "peace of mind", to be reasured that they do not have cancer, and that others go in the fear that a particular symptom means cancer and delay may permit it to spread. Certainly, no one goes with the hope or expectation of having cancer detected at any stage, early or otherwise. The test that is designed to reveal conditions that can be treated *before* they become true cancer will therefore tend to be more acceptable to the public; and so far not enough has been made of this aspect in some educational programmes.

Methods of Education

It should be said at once that there is no simple formula for effective public education about cancer. Every medium of publicity can be used, from the large-scale use of newspapers, films, and television to the more personal forms of persuasion exercised by doctors on their patients. There is no intrinsic merit in any one medium of publicity; it cannot be said that lectures are better than films, or that pamphlets are better than posters. All have their place in a properly designed programme of education. What can be said, however, is that studies in Canada, Britain and the U.S.A. (reviewed in WAKEFIELD, 1963) suggest strongly that the impersonal media of publicity (pamphlets, posters, films, etc.) are less effective than the personal media (lectures, discussions, personal advice, etc.) in influencing the individual to act. Curibusly, television programmes appear, from Canadian evidence, to fall into the category of person-to-person communications, inasmuch as they come into the home and family (PHILLIPS and TAYLOR, 1961).

Perhaps one of the most striking examples of how differently various segments of the population gather information on health matters (Fig. 5) emerged in a study by SANSOM, PINNOCK and WAKEFIELD (1971). The Figure is based on the social classification used for census purposes in Great Britain, but these classes are very similar to various forms of stratification in use in other countries, in that they largely reflect income, educational level, housing, and so on. For instance, the women who were the subject of the study, described later, by FULGHUM (1967) and his colleagues in the U.S.A., would clearly be, in the British system of classification, members of class V, the wives of unskilled manual workers very low on the economic scale. The findings are neither new nor unique. They constitute a recurrent problem of public health and disease control: that often the people most at risk and most in need of preventive and detection measures make least use of these measures and are least able to respond to massive propaganda. The lower on the socio–economic scale, the more they rely on word-of-mouth for acceptable information, and least of all on large-scale publicity. A reverse gradient applies the higher up the scale we go.

There is little doubt that the most powerful *potential* influence of all is that of the physician in his direct relationship with his patients (MARTIN, 1964; KEGELES, KIRSCHT, HAEFNER and ROSENSTOCK, 1965; WAKEFIELD, 1972). He is often able to persuade them to accept examinations that they might never seek of their own accord, whereas the educationalist still has to find ways of getting apparently healty people to visit a doctor. A Gallup survey of a national sample for the American Cancer Society showed that 43% of women who had undergone cervical cytological examination had been influenced by their doctors. In other surveys, the proportion was even greater—as high as 90% in a survey in Alameda County, California (BRESLOW and HOCHSTIM, 1964). The powerful effect of personal persuasion by nurses and social workers was also revealed in the Dade County, Florida, project (FULGHUM, 1967). This study was particularly interesting in that it was concerned with a high-risk group of women very low on the socio–economic scale. More recently in England, OSBORN and LEYSHON (1966) described a local project in which public health nurses used their special local knowledge to select

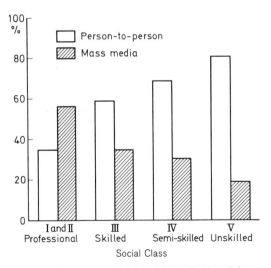

Fig. 5. How women of each social class first heard about the cervical smear test. (Survey of 200 women examined by family doctor)

and persuade high-risk women, *and* took cervical smears in their homes. They examined 783 women and claimed an incidence of carcinoma *in situ* of 26.5 per 1,000—almost four times the incidence in the population at large and among the women voluntarily visiting the town's cytology clinic.

More recently, GALLUP (1974), in a sample survey of 1,007 women for the American Cancer Society in 1973 of women's attitudes to breast cancer, investigated the extent to which the Society's long advocacy of breast self-examination had succeeded. Awareness of this procedure was high among the sample (77%), but few (18%) had practised it regularly over the preceding year. It is in the sources of their information that particular interest lies: 32% had learned about it from a physician, compared with 17% from magazine articles, 8% television, 8% newspapers, 2% radio, and 6% from pamphlets not obtained from a physician. The report said that in persuading women to act, "the mass media are measurably less effective when it comes to actual practice... Since physicians are particularly effective in translating mere awareness of breast self-examination into actual practice, it is unfortunate that more do not make a greater effort to familiarize women with it."

This is not intended as an argument for or against this particular form of detection measure: it is simply another example of the large responsibility that rests with doctors in the matter of persuasion and education. Whether they like it or not, their every word, gesture or facial expression is a form of public education. The only question is whether its effect will be for good or ill. They are, in the main, unaware of their potential in this matter and, in most countries, untrained for it. This is not the place for a lengthy treatment on professional education. However, it needs to be said with great emphasis that the training of doctors is still deficient on two counts: (1) the amount of attention devoted to the detection of early malignant diesease; and (2) the treatment of the doctor's

role, voluntary or involuntary, in the education of his patients. The same can be said for the training of all nurses and other paramedical workers who come into contact with cancer patients. The public sees them as sources of expert knowledge, however ill-equipped they may be, with particular information about cancer.

Against the undoubted effectiveness of person-to-person communication, we must set the difficulty and expense of reaching a wide public by such means. Although conversation and gossip are known to spread personal messages widely by the so-called "ripple effect", there is usually no alternative to the mass media in spreading information widely throughout the population. Although the mass media may be less obviously effective in persuading individuals to take action, they can do much to create a climate of greater receptivity to the more personal forms of persuasion. And since cancer is still a "taboo" subject in many communities, thoughtful and well-planned publicity on a large scale can do much to break down barriers to free discussion, to transfer cancer in the public mind from its position of special dread to the more reasonable status of one of the serious but manageable diseases of today. The extent to which cancer is still believed to be always incurable is alarming (UICC Monograph series, No. 5). Altering this belief is one of the prime objectives of any cancer education programme; for until people believe that treatment will help them, they see no urgency in seeking medical advice and no purpose in early diagnosis. That it *can* be done has been demonstrated convincingly in Canada and the U.S.A. (by 1962, only 12.3% of a U.S. national-survey sample still thought that cancer could never be cured).

It should be made clear, however, that the media of publicity are merely the tools of the educator. It is possible to go to great expense to produce films or pamphlets that fail because of shortcomings in the information or the way in which it is expressed.

Health educators are very prone to becoming involved in the technicalities of their work, and in spending much time and energy in devising new ways of using old tools. Of course technical expertise is required, but we should remember that the basic way of communicating is by the spoken or written word, whether by individuals, newspapers, film, or television. The extent to which one medium or another should be used will depend entirely on local conditions, which vary enormously from one country to another.

Social Conditions and Cancer Detection

Even more important in designing programmes of education is awareness that beliefs about cancer and accepted patterns of behaviour in health and disease are extremely varied. It is not even always possible to talk of national patterns of behaviour, since what is accepted as normal may vary within the same country and from one social or economic group to another. Rural communities generally tend toward the stoical view of accepting a person as "sick" only when he is quite unable to work any longer; middle-class urban communities are more likely to accept preventive checks and prompt medical care, for even minor ailments, as normal and proper. Economic deprivation also fosters a reluctance to admit illness and the consequent inability to continue earning.

These are not, of course, the only factors that bear on the willingness or reluctance of people to participate in cancer detection programmes; we simply offer them as examples of the kind of sociological information required before an adequate programme of education can be devised. It is pointless, for example, to expect education about preventive health measures, or even early detection, to have any quick effect on a community which regards "calling in the doctor" as the ultimate confession of weakness. In the past, health education programmes of many kinds have failed because they began without adequate information about the people they were intended to serve. Too often, these programmes have been based on "common sense", which usually refers to what the middle-class professional educator thinks he knows about his own people. Unfortunately, his standards and beliefs are often far removed from those of his countrymen further down the educational or economic scale, and the inevitable result is a failure of communication. The educator is puzzled by the "irrational" attitudes of those he is seeking to educate, and he takes refuge in labelling those who do not respond to his message as "resistant", "hard-to-reach", or "unintelligent". Yet people always have reason for acting as they do. To a man who is on the verge of poverty or who is insecure in his job, any test designed to reveal a serious disease is seen, with good reason, as a threat to his precarious way of life. He is concerned with geting through today, not planning for the future; and he simply does not understand the middle-class preoccupation with planning ahead, be it in matters of finance or good health.

The varied responses from people of different educational and economic status emerged very clearly in recent studies of cytological screening programmes for uterine cancer in Britain (MACGREGOR and BAIRD, 1963; WAKEFIELD and BARIĆ, 1965; WAKEFIELD, 1972) and the U.S.A. (BRESLOW and HOCHSTIM, 1964; Gallup survey, 1964; KEGELES et al., 1965). The Gallup survey showed a response rate of 63% among women in the group with the highest income level, but only 28% in those with the lowest. The range was similar between women with college education (63%) and grade school education (35%). In the Alameda County survey, the response ranged from 63% in social class I to 36% in social class V. In each instance, the lowest response is found among women in the groups which are most at risk.

However, that those lowest on the social scale are not inherently unresponsive or resistant to education was shown by FULGHUM'S (1967) investigation in Florida, U.S.A., of women low on the social and economic scale, who had not responded to earlier invitations to participate in a screening programme. It revealed unspoken fears about the nature and outcome of the Papanicolaou test, a "functional illiteracy" that hindered the women from responding to printed· publicity, and a complex network by which communications were spread and accepted throughout the community. Subsequent educational programmes directed at similar women in other parts of Florida were based on these findings, in one county, over 72% of the target population had the examination (ANNE ROLFE, personal communication)—a response better than that of the higher social classes of most other studies. In fact, when response is poor, the communication is often at fault, not the recipients. It can also be that administrative and bureaucratic barriers to participation arise unnoticed, hampering action by those whom education has successfully motivated (WAKEFIELD, 1972; VUORI et al., 1972).

One point should be made clear, however: although the response rate is least favourable among people lowest on the social and economic scale, there are substantial numbers from all the social classes who do not participate. Of those who *do* respond,

the proportion of people who return for subsequent examination at regular intervals is depressingly small. Here is one area in which research is urgently needed, since most of our present information concerns those who have undergone examination. We know very little about the reasons why people decide not to participate. However, a survey in Western Australia showed that, of the people who had never had a cancer examination, it was the women over 60 years old and the single, divorced, separated, and widowed women who were most reluctant to consider having one. The same pattern emerged in a 10-year series of studies in England (WAKEFIELD, 1972). This suggests an interesting area for research: Is the influence of men an important factor in motivating women to undergo examination? If so, the implications for public education would be interesting; information about cancer-detection examinations for women would have to be aimed specifically at their menfolk, as well as at the women themselves. We also know little about why those who have been examined once decide not to return for further examinations at regular intervals. A recent study by SANSOM, MCINERNEY, and OLIVER (in preparation) showed that practical difficulties and organizational flaws were at least as important as unfortunate initial experiences, and that tests done as an adjunct to another vaginal examination were often not understood by the woman to be special procedures that needed to be repeated at intervals (SANSOM, WAKEFIELD and PINNOCK, 1971).

Research and Evaluation

Until some of these gaps in our knowledge are filled, we shall not be able to make our educational programmes as effective as they might be, for we cannot be sure we are getting to the root of the problem. One of the commonest mistakes in health education has been to assume that when a programme is not as effective as expected, not

enough time, money, or energy has been spent on it. But if a programme is based on inadequate data or its content is unsuitable, it can never be improved by merely increasing the dose; it simply becomes a failure on a greater scale. It is equally true that adequate preparatory work and elegant design are powerless unless they are geared to the driving force of organizational skills, money and personal effort.

It is regrettable that the need for research into the effectiveness of educational methods and of the results of programmes is rarely accorded the priority it needs. Driving force and prodigious human effort cannot automatically be equated with achievement. Faith that what we are doing *must* be right because it is directed against cancer is laudable, but not enough. The effort, however massive, may be misdirected, the money unwisely used. We simply cannot tell unless measurement and evaluation are built into the educational programme from the outset.

Like all scientific evaluation, this effort requires that we precisely define the aims of the educational programme before it begins. Without such definition, honest measurement is later impossible. Questions may be asked, such as: Is the aim to persuade poorly educated countrywomen to attend a mobile gynaecological clinic? Or, are we striving to persuade an adequate proportion of women over the age of 50 to attend regularly for mammographic examination (or palpation, or both) at specified intervals? Later, the extent to which these aims have been achieved can and should be measured. Here, a note of caution is necessary: the target set for the educationalist is not necessarily identical to that of the oncologist. Everyone in cancer control is aiming to achieve the detection of more cancers at a treatable stage. But this is a broad, general aim that is the desired end-product of the efforts of many different people, lay and professional. The educator needs more sharply defined targets; even then, the measure of his success or failure is not that which his clinical colleagues would apply. We could say, for instance, that the aim of an educational programme is to teach all women in a region that post-menopausal bleeding always requires medical investigation. The clinician's ultimate aim is to detect early cancers in such women; he measures success by detecting a larger number of such cases than are found in similar regions without an educational programme. But the educationalist, though part of the team dedicated to detecting early cancer, has achieved *his* objective when *any* post-menopausal women with bleeding see a doctor. His educational message has been successful, regardless of whether the subsequent diagnosis is malignancy or not. This is not mere hair-splitting: it is an expression of the need for clear thinking on what we expect education to achieve. For a fuller treatment of evaluation in cancer education, readers are referred to the publication Health Education: Theory and Practice in Cancer Control (1974), Vol. 10, in the UICC Technical Report Series.

In addition to the evaluation of results there are other areas for research. For instance, we lack adequate sociological and psychological information on whether it is better to offer a number of tests at the same time, or each one singly. The proportion of women in the United States who have had a Papanicolaou test has risen steadily since 1960, whereas the proportion of the general population who have had a complete annual physical has recently remained static. In other words, the single preventive test seems to be more readily accepted than a battery of tests. REZNIKOFF (1955) in the United States investigated some of the important factors involved in motivating people to visit a cancer detection centre for a complete checkup. "Cancer among close relatives, a history of serious illness, and emotional difficulties... and apprehension were very prevalent" in the group of 100 people he studied. There is evidence from one small study in Rotherham, England, that people preferred to go for a battery of health tests (which included a chest X-ray and cervical cytology) than to go for any one of these tests alone. But it should be noted that the other simple tests were for non-malignant diseases, and people probably found it easier to accept what was ostensibly a general health check-up than to make the decision to go for a specific examination for one feared disease. We may have to be prepared to accept that, even when medical facilities are available in every country, the complete "cancer checkup" will not be accepted widely enough by *all* sections of the community to have any measurable effect on mortality figures. Perhaps when treatment is demonstrably effective for all forms of cancer (as when streptomycin changed the whole public attitude toward TB), cancer tests will be more acceptable psychologically. But meanwhile, cancer is still widely regarded as a single incurable disease; the concept of a family of related diseases, some highly curable, some very difficult or impossible to cure, is not yet a familiar one in all countries. All forms of cancer are therefore seen in the melancholy light of those with the worst prognosis; and to be told they have cancer is for most people a sentence of death with no possibility of reprieve. In this climate of opinion, what possible attraction can there be in going to a doctor for a series of examinations, some of them uncomfortable, in order to learn one's death sentence a little sooner than otherwise? This is how the situation looks to many laymen who do not share the enthusiasm of the medical men and health educators for these new tests; and we cannot expect to win general acceptance for regular screening until the background of accurate general knowledge about cancer in all levels of the community has been brought to the point where the advantages of early detection and treatment become self-evident.

It is important, therefore, not to divorce publicity on specific programmes of detection from the wider context of public education about the increasingly hopeful outlook for many forms of cancer. This comment may seem trite in countries which have long-established programmes of cancer education and detection. But in countries with large high-risk populations, where the benefits of introducing, for example, cytotests for uterine cancer seem so attractive, there is a real danger that too much attention will be devoted to publicizing the test without regard to the reassuring background of infor-

mation needed to make the test acceptable to the women most in need of it. (Will the test interfere with normal sex-life? Will it reveal past misdemeanours? Will it cause sterility? Will whatever is found be curable?) These are all typical questions which, because they went unanswered, have caused women to be reluctant in the past.

Public acceptance of a detection test is a matter that has not always received adequate attention in the planning of public education. Painstaking research and testing in the hospital setting may prove beyond doubt the effectiveness of a particular form of cancer detection examination; but no amount of publicity and medical enthusiasm will convince large numbers of the general public (as distinguished from the health-conscious minority) to accept the examination if they find it notably unpleasant or distasteful. The possibility of discovering and removing a possible threat to future well-being will never have as high a priority as the negative motivation of an unpleasant procedure. And those who try a new test once, even a comparatively innocuous one such as cervical cytology, sometimes find it distasteful enough to discourage repetition. How much greater, then, is the problem of persuading large numbers of people to accept an examination such as proctoscopy, which has been shown to be very useful as a means of cancer detection? However, it is a big jump from proving its effectiveness to persuading the man in the street to overcome his deep natural revulsion against the procedure involved. HAMMERSCHLAG (1952) summarized the psychological barriers that make ano-rectal examination peculiarly difficult to accept, even when an individual has obvious symptoms to justify the examination. This may seem an unduly pessimistic view of the chances of incorporating regular proctoscopic examination into programmes of cancer detection. However, it is intended, rather, as an attempt to show that responsibility for "selling" a medically desirable test to the public cannot be placed entirely upon the educationalist and publicist. We must recognize that there are limits to what the educationalist can do, just as there are limits to what the surgeon can do. If a test involves inevitable discomfort or arouses revulsion, there is little likelihood that it will be accepted routinely by most of the people, however persuasive the educator may be. For people to take part in preventive health programmes, they must normally see the threat of the disease to *themselves* as far outweighing the present disadvantages or discomforts of taking the preventive test, and they must believe the test to be truly protective or the treatment wholly effective. HOCHBAUM (1959) and ROSENSTOCK (1961, 1969) have discussed preventive health behaviour in detail. Their models are valuable aids in the discussion of this difficult problem, though they should be recognized as broad generalizations, which the quirks and eccentricities of human behaviour do much to nullify. No general model can help us predict how various individuals will react to a disconcerting situation.

To summarize, what is required is public education that will: (1) provide a general background of hopeful information about cancer, emphasizing those forms for which cure is probable if treatment is started at an early stage, but making no exaggerated claims regarding the less manageable forms. This kind of information is necessary if detection tests are to be seen in true perspective, as a means of ensuring that people do not die needlessly of curable forms of cancer; (2) provide specific information about detection tests and what facilities are available for all sections of the population at risk. Determining which arguments are most persuasive depends entirely on the national and local characteristics of the people addressed and their values regarding health and disease. Discovering the nature of these beliefs is a prerequisite to successful education; they have to be identified before we can plan to change them. We also have to be acquainted with the barriers to public acceptance of detection tests before we can hope to devise appeals persuasive enough to overcome them. The rewards that come from winning public acceptance go beyond the immediate saving of life by early detection: every cancer or precancerous condition that is dealt with at a stage when treatment is least drastic will help considerably to diminish the spectre of cancer as the relentless killer.

References

BRESLOW, L., HOCHSTIM, J.R.: Sociocultural aspects of cervical cytology in Alameda County. Calif. Publ. Hlth Rep. **79**, 107–112 (1964).

FULGHUM, J.E.: Cervical cancer detection through cytology (Monograph Series, No. 11). Jacksonville: Florida State Board of Health 1967.

HAMMERSCHLAG, E.: Psychiatry applied to internal medicine. In: Bellak, L. (ed.), Psychology of physical illness. London: Churchill Ltd. 1952.

HOCHBAUM, G.M.: Public participation in medical screening programs: a socio-psychological study. U.S. Public Health Service Pubn. 572 (1958).

KEGELES, S.S., KIRSCHT, J.P., HAEFNER, D.P., ROSENSTOCK, I.M.: Sruvey of beliefs about cancer detection and taking Papanicolaou tests. Publ. Hlth Rep. **80**, 815–823 (1965).

MACGREGOR, J.E., BAIRD, D.: Detection of cervical carcinoma in the general population. Brit. med. J. **1963**, 1631–1636.

MARTIN, P.L.: Detection of cervical cancer: A study of motivation for cytological screening. Calif. Med. **101**, 427–429 (1964).

OSBORN, G.R., LEYSHON, V.N.: Domiciliary testing of cervical smears by home nurses. Lancet **1966 I**, 256–257.

PHILLIPS, A.J., TAYLOR, R.M.: Public opinion on cancer in Canada: a second survey. Canad. med. Ass. J. **84**, 142–145 (1961).

The public's awareness and use of cancer detection tests. Conducted for the American Cancer Society by the Gallup Organization. Princeton, N.J. 1964.

REZNIKOFF, M.: Motivational factors in persons attending a cancerdetection center. Cancer (Philad.) **8**, 454–458 (1955).

ROLFE, A.: Personal communication.

ROSENSTOCK, I.M.: Decision-making by Individuals. Health Education Monographs No. 11, 1961.

ROSENSTOCK, I.M.: Health behaviour: Prevention and maintenance. In: Poverty and health, a sociological analysis, ed. by KOSA, J., ANTONOVSKY, A., ZOLA, I.K. Cambridge, Mass: Harvard Univ. Press 1969.

SANSOM, C.D., McINERNEY, J., OLIVER, V.: Differential response to recall in a cervical cytology programme. (in preparation).

SANSOM, C.D., WAKEFIELD, J., PINNOCK, K.M.: Choice or chance? How women come to have a cytotest done by their family doctors. Int. J. Hlth Educ. 2, 54 (1971).

Social survey of community attitudes to cancer: Metropolitan area of Perth, Western Australia. Research report Cancer Council of Western Australia. Perth: Univ. Western Australia 1965.

U.I.C.C. Monograph No. 5. Public education about Cancer: Research concepts the theoretical findings. Berlin-Heidelberg-New York: Springer 1967.

VUORI, H. RIMPÊLA, A., GRÖNROOS, M.: Cytological screening programmes: the problem of non-participation. Int. J. Hlth Educ. 15, 1 (1972).

WAKEFIELD, J.: Cancer and public education. London: Pitman Medical Publ. 1963.

WAKEFIELD, J. (ed.): Seek Wisely to Prevent. London: H.M.S.O. 1972.

WAKEFIELD, J., BARIĆ, L.: Public and professional attitudes to a screening programme for the prevention of cancer of the uterine cervix: a preliminary study. Brit. J. prev. soc. Med. 19, 151–158 (1965).

World Health Organization. Prevention of cancer: report of a WHO expert committee. WHO Techn. Rep. Ser. 276. Geneva 1964.

UICC Publications

Kaposi's Sarcoma. S. Karger AG., Basle (Switzerland) — New York (1963).

Cancer of the urinary bladder. S. Karger AG., Basle (Switzerland) — New York (1963).

Prognosis of malignant tumours of the breast. S. Karger AG., Basle (Switzerland) — New York (1963).

The lymphoreticular tumours in Africa. S. Karger AG., Basle (Switzerland) — New York (1964).

Cellular control mechanisms and cancer. Elsevier Publishing Company, Amsterdam — London — New York (1964).

Illustrated Tumor Nomenclature. Springer-Verlag Berlin — Heidelberg — New York (1965).

Structure and control of the melanocyte. Springer-Verlag Berlin — Heidelberg — New York (1966).

Public education about cancer; cancer education programmes in various countries. UICC, Geneva (1967).

Cancer incidence in five continents. Springer-Verlag Berlin — Heidelberg — New York (1966).

UICC Monograph Series

Vol. 1: Cancer of the nasopharynx. Munksgaard, Copenhagen (1967).

Vol. 2: Specific tumour antigens. Munksgaard, Copenhagen (1967).

Vol. 3: Choriocarcinoma. Springer-Verlag Berlin — Heidelberg — New York (1966).

Vol. 4: Cancer detection, 2nd edition. Springer-Verlag Berlin — Heidelberg — New York (1967).

Vol. 5: Public education about cancer; research findings and theoretical concepts. Springer-Verlag Berlin — Heidelberg — New York (1967).

Vol. 6: Mechanisms of Invasion in Cancer. Springer-Verlag Berlin — Heidelberg — New York (1967).

Vol. 7: Potential Carcinogenic Hazards from Drugs. Springer-Verlag Berlin — Heidelberg — New York (1967).

Vol. 8: Treatment of Burkitt's Tumour. Springer-Verlag Berlin — Heidelberg — New York (1967)

Vol. 9: Proceedings of the Ninth International Cancer congress — Congress Lectures and Official Speeches. Springer-Verlag Berlin — Heidelberg — New York (1967).

Vol. 10: Proceedings of the Ninth International Cancer Congress — Panel discussions. Springer-Verlag Berlin — Heidelberg — New York (1967).

Vol. 11: Ovarian Cancer. Springer-Verlag Berlin — Heidelberg — New York (1968).

Vol. 12: Thyroid Cancer. Springer-Verlag Berlin — Heidelberg — New York (1969).

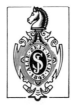